Editors

ASIF M. ILYAS
SHITAL N. PARIKH
SAQIB REHMAN
GILES R. SCUDERI
FELASFA M. WODAJO

ORTHOPEDIC CLINICS OF NORTH AMERICA

www.orthopedic.theclinics.com

April 2015 • Volume 46 • Number 2

ELSEVIER

1600 John F. Kennedy Boulevard • Suite 1800 • Philadelphia, Pennsylvania, 19103-2899.

http://www.orthopedic.theclinics.com

ORTHOPEDIC CLINICS OF NORTH AMERICA Volume 46, Number 2
April 2015 ISSN 0030-5898, ISBN-13: 978-0-323-35979-5

Editor: Jennifer Flynn-Briggs
Developmental Editor: Stephanie Wissler

Orthopedic Clinics of North America (ISSN 0030-5898) is published quarterly by Elsevier Inc., 360 Park Avenue South, New York, NY 10010-1710. Months of issue are January, April, July, and October. Business and Editorial Offices: 1600 John F. Kennedy Blvd., Suite 1800, Philadelphia, PA 19103-2899. Customer Service Office: 3251 Riverport Lane, Maryland Heights, MO 63043. Periodicals postage paid at New York, NY and additional mailing offices. Subscription prices are $310.00 per year for (US individuals), $596.00 per year for (US institutions), $365.00 per year (Canadian individuals), $727.00 per year (Canadian institutions), $450.00 per year (international individuals), $727.00 per year (international institutions), $150.00 per year (US students), $220.00 per year (Canadian and international students). Foreign air speed delivery is included in all *Clinics* subscription prices. All prices are subject to change without notice. **POSTMASTER:** Send change of address to *Orthopedic Clinics of North America*, **Elsevier Health Sciences Division, Subscription Customer Service, 3251 Riverport Lane, Maryland Heights, MO 63043. Customer Service (orders, claims, online, change of address): Elsevier Health Sciences Division, Subscription Customer Service, 3251 Riverport Lane, Maryland Heights, MO 63043. Tel: 1-800-654-2452 (U.S. and Canada); 314-447-8871 (outside U.S. and Canada). Fax: 314-447-8029. E-mail: journalscustomerservice-usa@elsevier. com (for print support); journalsonlinesupport-usa@elsevier.com (for online support).**

Reprints. For copies of 100 or more, of articles in this publication, please contact the Commercial Reprints Department, Elsevier Inc., 360 Park Avenue South, New York, NY 10010-1710. Tel.: 212-633-3874; Fax: 212-633-3820; E-mail: reprints@elsevier. com.

Orthopedic Clinics of North America is covered in *MEDLINE/PubMed* (*Index Medicus*), *Cinahl, Excerpta Medica,* and *Cumulative Index to Nursing and Allied Health Literature.*

PROGRAM OBJECTIVE

Orthopedic Clinics of North America offers clinical review articles on the most cutting-edge technologies and techniques in the field, including adult reconstruction, the upper extremity, pediatrics, trauma, oncology, and sports medicine.

TARGET AUDIENCE

Practicing orthopedic surgeons, orthopedic residents, and other healthcare professionals who specialize in orthopedic technologies and techniques for adult reconstruction, the upper extremity, pediatrics, trauma, oncology, and sports medicine.

LEARNING OBJECTIVES

Upon completion of this activity, participants will be able to:
1. Review treatments and wound care strategies in orthopaedic traumas.
2. Discuss the management of orthopaedic injuries of the upper extremity.
3. Recognize current trends in the treatments for hip and knee arthroplasty.

ACCREDITATION

The Elsevier Office of Continuing Medical Education (EOCME) is accredited by the Accreditation Council for Continuing Medical Education (ACCME) to provide continuing medical education for physicians.

The EOCME designates this enduring material for a maximum of 15 *AMA PRA Category 1 Credit*(s)™. Physicians should claim only the credit commensurate with the extent of their participation in the activity.

All other health care professionals requesting continuing education credit for this enduring material will be issued a certificate of participation.

DISCLOSURE OF CONFLICTS OF INTEREST

The EOCME assesses conflict of interest with its instructors, faculty, planners, and other individuals who are in a position to control the content of CME activities. All relevant conflicts of interest that are identified are thoroughly vetted by EOCME for fair balance, scientific objectivity, and patient care recommendations. EOCME is committed to providing its learners with CME activities that promote improvements or quality in healthcare and not a specific proprietary business or a commercial interest.

The planning committee, staff, authors and editors listed below have identified no financial relationships or relationships to products or devices they or their spouse/life partner have with commercial interest related to the content of this CME activity:

Irfan Ahmed, MD; Daniel M. Avery III, MD; Jared L. Braud, MD; Leonard T. Buller, MD; Nicholas M. Caggiano, MD; Stephanie Carter; Stephen M. Derrington, DO; Keith A. Fehring, MD; Jennifer Flynn-Briggs; Anjali Fortna; Mark J. Gage, MD; Ari C. Greis, DO; Marty Herman, MD; Robert E. Howell, MD; Brynne Hunter; Asif M. Ilyas, MD; Peter C. Krause, MD; Charles M. Lawrie, MD; Frank A. Liporace, MD; Matthew McAuliffe, MD; Jaydev Mistry, BS; Eric M. Padegimas, MD; Gurpal S. Pannu, MD; Nirav K. Pandya, MD; Shital N. Parikh, MD; Santha Priya; Mia Smucny, MD; Megan Suermann; Nathan J. Turnbull, MD; Fernando E. Vilella, MD; John M. Whatley, MD; Felasfa M. Wodajo, MD; Richard S. Yoon, MD.

The planning committee, staff, authors and editors listed below have identified financial relationships or relationships to products or devices they or their spouse/life partner have with commercial interest related to the content of this CME activity:

Keith R. Berend, MD is a consultant/advisor for, with a research grant and royalties/patents from Biomet, Inc., and has a research grant from Pacira Pharmaceuticals.

Kenneth A. Egol, MD is a consultant/advisor for, with royalties/patents from Exactech, Inc., as well as royalties/patents from Lippinocott and Slack Technologies, Inc.

Thomas K. Fehring, MD is a consultant/advisor for DePuy Synthes, with a research grant from DePuy Synthes and Johnson & Johnson Services, Inc.

Adolph V. Lombardi Jr, MD, FACS is on the speakers bureau for, a consultant/advisor for, and has research grants from Biomet, Inc., as well as research grants from Pacira Pharmaceuticals, Inc. and Innomed, Inc. He has royalties/patents from Biomet, Inc and Innomed, Inc.

Kristofer S. Matullo, MD is a consultant/advisor for DePuy Synthes.

Saqib Rehman, MD is on the speakers bureau for Synthes, Inc.

Giles R. Scuderi, MD is on the speakers bureau for, a consultant/advisor for, and has royalties/patents from Zimmer Inc. He is on the speakers bureau for, with a research grant from Pacira Pharmaceuticals, and on the speakers bureau for Medtronic and Convatec Inc.

UNAPPROVED/OFF-LABEL USE DISCLOSURE

The EOCME requires CME faculty to disclose to the participants:
1. When products or procedures being discussed are off-label, unlabelled, experimental, and/or investigational (not US Food and Drug Administration [FDA] approved); and
2. Any limitations on the information presented, such as data that are preliminary or that represent ongoing research, interim analyses, and/or unsupported opinions. Faculty may discuss information about pharmaceutical agents that is outside of

FDA-approved labelling. This information is intended solely for CME and is not intended to promote off-label use of these medications. If you have any questions, contact the medical affairs department of the manufacturer for the most recent prescribing information.

TO ENROLL

To enroll in the *Orthopedic Clinics of North America* Continuing Medical Education program, call customer service at 1-800-654-2452 or sign up online at http://www.theclinics.com/home/cme. The CME program is available to subscribers for an additional annual fee of USD $310.

METHOD OF PARTICIPATION

In order to claim credit, participants must complete the following:
1. Complete enrolment as indicated above.
2. Read the activity.
3. Complete the CME Test and Evaluation. Participants must achieve a score of 70% on the test. All CME Tests and Evaluations must be completed online.

CME INQUIRIES/SPECIAL NEEDS

For all CME inquiries or special needs, please contact elsevierCME@elsevier.com.

Contributors

EDITORS

ASIF M. ILYAS, MD - *Upper Extremity*
Program Director of Hand Surgery Fellowship,
Rothman Institute; Associate Professor of
Orthopaedic Surgery, Jefferson Medical
College, Philadelphia, Pennsylvania

SHITAL N. PARIKH, MD - *Pediatric
Orthopedics*
Pediatric Orthopaedics and Sports Trauma,
Associate Professor of Orthopaedic Surgery,
Cincinnati Children's Hospital Medical Center,
University of Cincinnati School of Medicine,
Cincinnati, Ohio

SAQIB REHMAN, MD - *Trauma*
Director of Orthopaedic Trauma, Associate
Professor of Orthopaedic Surgery and Sports
Medicine, School of Medicine, Temple
University Hospital, Temple University,
Philadelphia, Pennsylvania

GILES R. SCUDERI, MD - *Adult
Reconstruction*
Vice President, Orthopedic Service Line,
Northshore Long Island Jewish Health System;
Fellowship Director, Adult Knee
Reconstruction Lenox Hill Hospital, New York,
New York

FELASFA M. WODAJO, MD - *Oncology*
Musculoskeletal Tumor Surgery, Medical
Director, Musculoskeletal Oncology, Virginia
Hospital Center; Assistant Professor,
Orthopedic Surgery, Georgetown University
Hospital; Assistant Professor, Orthopedic
Surgery, VCU School of Medicine, Inova
Campus, Arlington, Virginia

AUTHORS

IRFAN AHMED, MD
Assistant Professor, Department of
Orthopedics, Rutgers University Hospital, New
Jersey Medical School, Newark, New Jersey

DANIEL M. AVERY III, MD
Department of Orthopaedic Surgery,
St. Luke's University Hospital, Bethlehem,
Pennsylvania

KEITH R. BEREND, MD
Joint Implant Surgeons, Inc., New Albany, Ohio

JARED L. BRAUD, MD
Orthopedic Surgery Resident, Department of
Orthopaedic Surgery, Louisiana State
University Health Sciences Center, New
Orleans, Louisiana

LEONARD T. BULLER, MD
Resident, Departments of Orthopaedic
Surgery and Rehabilitation, Jackson Memorial
Hospital, University of Miami, Miami, Florida

NICHOLAS M. CAGGIANO, MD
Department of Orthopaedic Surgery, St. Luke's
University Hospital, Bethlehem, Pennsylvania

STEPHEN M. DERRINGTON, DO
Department of Physical Medicine and
Rehabilitation, Thomas Jefferson University,
Philadelphia, Pennsylvania

KENNETH A. EGOL, MD
Vice Chairman, Division of Orthopaedic
Trauma, Department of Orthopaedic Surgery,
NYU Hospital for Joint Diseases, New York,
New York

KEITH A. FEHRING, MD
Adult Reconstruction Fellow, Department of
Orthopaedic Surgery, Mayo Clinic, Rochester,
Minnesota

THOMAS K. FEHRING, MD
Co-director, Ortho Carolina Hip and Knee
Center, Charlotte, North Carolina

MARK J. GAGE, MD
Resident, Division of Orthopaedic Trauma,
Department of Orthopaedic Surgery, NYU
Hospital for Joint Diseases, New York,
New York

ARI C. GREIS, DO
Clinical Instructor, Department of Physical
Medicine and Rehabilitation, Rothman
Institute, Thomas Jefferson University,
Philadelphia, Pennsylvania

MARTY HERMAN, MD
Department of Orthopedic Surgery and
Pediatrics, Drexel University College of
Medicine, Philadelphia, Pennsylvania

ROBERT E. HOWELL, MD
Joint Implant Surgeons, Inc., New Albany,
Ohio

ASIF M. ILYAS, MD
Program Director of Hand Surgery
Fellowship, Rothman Institute; Associate
Professor of Orthopaedic Surgery,
Jefferson Medical College, Philadelphia,
Pennsylvania

PETER C. KRAUSE, MD
Associate Professor, Department of
Orthopaedic Surgery, Louisiana State
University Health Sciences Center, New
Orleans, Louisiana

CHARLES M. LAWRIE, MD
Resident, Departments of Orthopaedic
Surgery and Rehabilitation, Jackson
Memorial Hospital, University of Miami,
Miami, Florida

FRANK A. LIPORACE, MD
Director, Orthopaedic Trauma Research,
Associate Professor, Division of Orthopaedic
Trauma, Department of Orthopaedic Surgery,
NYU Hospital for Joint Diseases, New York,
New York; Vice Chair and Chief, Orthopaedic

Trauma and Adult Reconstruction, Department
of Orthopaedic Surgery, Jersey City Medical
Center, Jersey City, New Jersey

ADOLPH V. LOMBARDI Jr, MD, FACS
Joint Implant Surgeons, Inc., New Albany,
Ohio

KRISTOFER S. MATULLO, MD
Chief, Division of Hand Surgery,
Department of Orthopaedic Surgery,
St. Luke's University Health Network,
Bethlehem, Pennsylvania

MATTHEW McAULIFFE, MD
Department of Physical Medicine and
Rehabilitation, Thomas Jefferson University,
Philadelphia, Pennsylvania

JAYDEV MISTRY, BS
Rutgers University Hospital, New Jersey
Medical School, Newark, New Jersey

ERIC M. PADEGIMAS, MD
Resident Physician, Department of
Orthopaedic Surgery, Thomas Jefferson
University Hospital, Philadelphia,
Pennsylvania

NIRAV K. PANDYA, MD
Assistant Professor, Department of
Orthopaedic Surgery, University of California
San Francisco Benioff Children's Hospital
Oakland, Oakland, California

GURPAL S. PANNU, MD
Department of Orthopedic Surgery and
Pediatrics, Drexel University College of
Medicine, Philadelphia, Pennsylvania

SHITAL N. PARIKH, MD
Pediatric Orthopaedics and Sports Trauma,
Associate Professor of Orthopaedic Surgery,
Cincinnati Children's Hospital Medical Center,
University of Cincinnati School of Medicine,
Cincinnati, Ohio

MIA SMUCNY, MD
Resident, Department of Orthopaedic Surgery,
University of California San Francisco,
San Francisco, California

NATHAN J. TURNBULL, MD
Joint Implant Surgeons, Inc., New Albany,
Ohio

FERNANDO E. VILELLA, MD
Assistant Professor, Orthopaedic Trauma
Service, Department of Orthopaedic
Surgery, Ryder Trauma Center, Jackson
Memorial Hospital, University of Miami,
Miami, Florida

JOHN M. WHATLEY, MD
Orthopedic Surgery Resident,
Department of Orthopaedic Surgery,
Louisiana State University Health
Sciences Center, New Orleans,
Louisiana

FELASFA M. WODAJO, MD
Musculoskeletal Tumor Surgery, Medical
Director, Musculoskeletal Oncology, Virginia
Hospital Center; Assistant Professor,
Orthopedic Surgery, Georgetown University
Hospital; Assistant Professor, Orthopedic
Surgery, VCU School of Medicine, Inova
Campus, Arlington, Virginia

RICHARD S. YOON, MD
Resident, Division of Orthopaedic Trauma,
Department of Orthopaedic Surgery, NYU
Hospital for Joint Diseases, New York, New York

Contributors

FERNANDO E. VILELLA, MD
Assistant Professor, Orthopaedic Trauma
Service, Department of Orthopaedic
Surgery, Ryder Trauma Center, Jackson
Memorial Hospital, University of Miami,
Miami, Florida

JOHN M. WHATLEY, MD
Orthopaedic Surgery Resident,
Department of Orthopaedic Surgery,
Louisiana State University Health
Sciences Center, New Orleans,
Louisiana

FELASFA M. WODAJO, MD
Musculoskeletal Tumor Surgery, Medical
Director, Musculoskeletal Oncology, Virginia
Hospital Center; Assistant Professor,
Orthopedic Surgery, Georgetown University
Hospital; Assistant Professor, Orthopedic
Surgery, VCU School of Medicine, Inova
Campus, Arlington, Virginia

RICHARD S. YOON, MD
Resident, Division of Orthopaedic Trauma
Department of Orthopaedic Surgery, NYU
Hospital for Joint Diseases, New York, New York

Contents

Acetabular fractures in the elderly are most frequently the result of low-energy trauma and present unique management challenges to orthopedic surgeons. Evaluation and treatment should be performed in a multidisciplinary fashion with early involvement of internal medicine subspecialists and geriatricians. Distinct fracture patterns and pre-existing osteoarthritis and osteoporosis necessitate careful preoperative planning. The role of total hip arthroplasty should also be considered when surgical treatment is indicated. The outcomes of acetabular fractures in the elderly have improved, but complications remain higher and results less satisfactory than in younger individuals. The lack of randomized controlled trials has limited the ability to establish an evidence-based treatment algorithm.

Negative pressure wound therapy (NPWT) is a useful management tool in the treatment of traumatic wounds and high-risk incisions after surgery. Since its development nearly 2 decades ago, uses and indications of NPWT have expanded, allowing its use in a variety of clinical scenarios. In addition to providing a brief summary on its mechanism of action, this article provides a focused, algorithmic approach on the use of NPWT by reviewing the available data, the appropriate clinical scenarios and indications, and the specific strategies that can be used to maximize outcomes.

Pediatric Orthopaedics

Fractures involving the distal radius and ulna are commonly seen in children and adolescents. Management of these injuries in pediatric patients should include assessment of the neurovascular status of the extremity, associated soft-tissue injury, and, most importantly, possible involvement of the physes of the radius and ulna. Treatment of these injuries may vary from simple casting and radiographic follow-up to urgent reduction and surgical fixation. Regardless of the initial treatment plan, the treating surgeon must remain aware of the potential for both early and late complications that may affect outcomes.

Pediatric and adolescent sports participation has increased with a concomitant increase in injuries. Sports have transitioned from recreational to deliberate, structured activities wherein success is determined by achievement of 'elite' status. This has led to specialization in a single sport with intensive, repetitive activity at younger ages causing physical and emotional consequences, particularly true for the growing athlete who is particularly susceptible to injury. Clinicians caring for this population must understand the epidemiology of youth sports specialization, the unique physiology/structure of this age group, and the potential physical and emotional consequences.

Upper Extremity

Musculoskeletal injuries are the second most common cause of presentation to emergency departments. Distal radius fractures are an especially common injury pattern that often require evaluation and fracture management in an emergency department. This article reviews the evaluation of distal radius fractures including physical examination and radiographic review. Also discussed is management of distal radius fractures including splinting in the setting of an emergency department consultation.

Elbow dislocations are common injuries in both the adult and pediatric populations. These injuries include simple dislocation with no associated fracture and more complex injuries with bony and ligamentous involvement. Simple dislocations are generally stable after reduction and managed with early mobilization. Complex dislocations are very unstable and operative intervention is usually necessary. Complication risks are greater and outcomes are less optimal with complex dislocations. A thorough knowledge of anatomy and understanding of the osseous and soft tissue mechanics is essential for proper management of these injuries.

Injuries to the thumb ulnar collateral ligament (UCL) are common. Failure to address the ensuing laxity of the metacarpophalangeal joint can lead to compromised grip and pinch, pain, and ultimately osteoarthritis. Instability to valgus stress with the lack of a firm end point is a strong indicator of complete rupture of the UCL. Nonoperative treatment is reserved for incomplete ruptures of the thumb UCL. Operative intervention is typically performed for complete ruptures. Repair of acute ruptures and reconstruction for chronic injuries yield excellent results. Complications are rare and most patients show preservation of motion, key pinch, and grip strength.

Rotator cuff calcific tendinopathy is a common finding that accounts for about 7% of patients with shoulder pain. There are numerous theories on the pathogenesis of rotator cuff calcific tendinopathy. The diagnosis is confirmed with radiography, MRI or ultrasound. There are numerous conservative treatment options available and most patients can be managed successfully without surgical intervention. Nonsteroidal anti-inflammatory drugs and multiple modalities are often used to manage pain and inflammation; physical therapy can help improve scapular mechanics and decrease dynamic impingement; ultrasound-guided needle aspiration and lavage techniques can provide long-term improvement in pain and function in these patients.

Oncology

Patients with potential bone and soft tissue tumors can be challenging for orthopedic surgeons. Lesions that appear benign can still create anxiety for the clinician and patient. However, attention to a few key imaging and clinical findings is enough to correctly diagnose five of the most common bone and soft tissue lesions: lipoma, enchondroma, osteochondroma, nonossifying fibroma, and Paget disease. Accurate identification of these lesions should be within the scope of most orthopedic surgeons and, because most of these patients will not need surgical treatment, referral to orthopedic oncology will not typically be required.

ORTHOPEDIC CLINICS OF NORTH AMERICA

FORTHCOMING ISSUES

Beginning with the July 2013 issue, *Orthopedic Clinics of North America* began to appear in this new format. Rather than focusing on a single topic, each issue contains articles on key areas in orthopedics—adult reconstruction, upper extremity, trauma, pediatrics and oncology. Articles on sports medicine and foot and ankle will also be included on a regular basis. As the practice of orthopedics has become more specialized, the format of one topic per issue is no longer fulfilling our readers' needs. The new format is intended to address these changing needs.

Orthopedic Clinics of North America continues to publish a print issue four times a year, in January, April, July, and October. However, this series also includes online-only articles that will be published on a rolling basis (not in accordance with our quarterly publication dates). These articles, along with articles from our print issues, are available on http://www.orthopedic.theclinics.com/.

YOUR iPhone and iPad

Adult Reconstruction

Preface
Adult Reconstruction

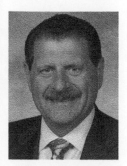

Giles R. Scuderi, MD
Editor

In this issue of *Orthopedic Clinics of North America*, we cover two current and relevant topics in joint arthroplasty: lateral unicompartmental knee arthroplasty and metal-on-metal total hip arthroplasty. In the first article by Berend and coauthors, it becomes apparent that while osteoarthritis affects the knee in a significant amount of the population, not all degenerative arthritis affects more than one compartment of the knee. In fact, isolated medial compartment arthritis is seen in approximately 25% of the affected population, while isolated lateral compartment disease is seen in 5% to 10% of patients. It is in this later group of patients with lateral compartment arthritis that the authors report on their clinical experience with isolated lateral unicompartmental knee arthroplasty. It is their observation that this approach is associated with less morbidity, a more rapid recovery, and more normal knee kinematics. With the limited number of reports on lateral unicompartmental knee arthroplasty, this article enhances the literature with a focus on patient selection, implant selection, and surgical technique.

The second article focuses on total hip arthroplasty (THA) and the modes of failure with metal-on-metal designs. In the last decade, metal-on-metal THA made resurgence with an expectation of improved wear, improved longevity, and lower dislocation rates. However, in recent years, new modes of failure, such as adverse local tissue reaction, with these bearings have been identified. In the article by Fehring and Fehring, the authors report on the modes of failure with metal-on-metal THA and discuss the evaluation and treatment modes of failure unique to this implant design. When evaluating a patient with a painful THA, the authors stress that it is important to consider all common modes of failure associated with conventional THA, in addition to the modes of failure unique to metal-on-metal THA. A systematic approach to these patients involves a careful history, physical examination, serology tests, and both radiographic and advanced imaging. Based on the findings of these multiple diagnostic variables, a treatment plan can be determined.

Both of these articles provide the reader with valuable insight on two different but contemporary topics in joint arthroplasty. Knowing that reading provides the mind with knowledge, I believe that these articles will be useful references.

Giles R. Scuderi, MD
Orthopedic Service Line
Northshore Long Island Jewish Health System
210 East 64th Street
New York, NY 10065, USA

E-mail address:
gscuderi@nshs.edu

http://dx.doi.org/10.1016/j.ocl.2014.12.005
0030-5898/15/$ – see front matter © 2015 Published by Elsevier Inc.

orthopedic.theclinics.com

The Current Trends for Lateral Unicondylar Knee Arthroplasty

Keith R. Berend, MD*, Nathan J. Turnbull, MD,
Robert E. Howell, MD, Adolph V. Lombardi Jr, MD

KEYWORDS

- Unicompartmental osteoarthritis • Unicondylar knee arthroplasty • Lateral • Osteoarthritis

KEY POINTS

- Osteoarthritis isolated to the lateral compartment occurs in 5% to 10% of individuals with osteoarthritis of the knee.
- Varus stress radiographs are critical to identifying patients with isolated lateral compartment osteoarthritis.
- The fact that the lateral compartment of the knee is looser in flexion than in extension must be taken into consideration when balancing the knee.
- Fixed-bearing implants have a better track record in lateral unicondylar knee replacement.
- With proper patient selection, implant choice, and surgical technique, the lateral unicondylar knee replacement has excellent results and early survivorship.

INTRODUCTION

Osteoarthritis affecting the knee causes a significant burden on society affecting 37.4% of people 45 years of age and older and 47.8% of those 60 years of age and older.[1,2] Severe tricompartmental disease is typically treated with a total knee arthroplasty (TKA), and the estimated cost associated with those hospitalizations was $28.5 in 2009.[3] The number of TKAs performed each year is rising and is projected to hit 3.8 million procedures per year by the year 2030.[4] However, not all degenerative joint disease affects more than one compartment.

Various studies report the rate of unicompartmental disease from 6% to 40%. Isolated medial compartment disease is seen in approximately 25% of knees with osteoarthritis, whereas isolated lateral compartment disease is only seen in 5% to 10%.[5] Historically, femoral and tibial osteotomies have been somewhat effective in treating

Disclosures: Keith R. Berend, Royalties, Consultant, Speaker's Bureau: Biomet, Inc. Institutional Research Support: Biomet, Inc., Stryker, Kinamed, Pacira; Piedmont Orthopaedic Society. Investment Interest: VuMedi.com. Publications editorial board: Clinical Orthopaedics and Related Research, Journal of Arthroplasty, Journal of Bone and Joint Surgery American, Orthopedics, Reconstructive Review. Board member/committee appointment: The Knee Society, American Association of Hip and Knee Surgeons, Board of Specialty Societies.
Adolph V. Lombardi Jr, Consultant, Speaker's Bureau: Biomet, Inc.; Pacira. Royalties: Biomet, Inc.; Innomed, Inc. Research Support: Biomet, Inc.; Stryker; Pacira; Kinamed. Publications Editorial Boards: Journal of Arthroplasty; Journal of Bone and Joint Surgery - American; Clinical Orthopaedics and Related Research; Journal of the American Academy of Orthopaedic Surgeons; Journal of Orthopaedics and Traumatology; Surgical Technology International; The Knee. Boards: Operation Walk USA; The Hip Society; The Knee Society; Mount Carmel Education Center at New Albany
Joint Implant Surgeons, Inc. 7277 Smith's Mill Road, Suite 200, New Albany, OH 43054, USA
* Corresponding author.
E-mail address: BerendKR@joint-surgeons.com

Orthop Clin N Am 46 (2015) 177–184
http://dx.doi.org/10.1016/j.ocl.2014.10.001

unicompartmental disease that does not involve full-thickness cartilage lesions; however, they have not been effective in cases with full-thickness lesions.

Unicondylar knee arthroplasty (UKA), as opposed to TKA, provides a less invasive, more conservative option to patients with osteoarthritis affecting only one of the three compartments of the knee. Studies have shown that UKA has reduced associated morbidity, a more rapid recovery, more preserved bone stock, more physiologically normal kinematics, and better postoperative range of motion compared with TKA. In addition, UKA feels closer to a native knee and has a more normal gait pattern.[5]

Data suggest that UKA is not always being performed when indicated. Medial UKA and lateral UKA constitutes only 11% (10% and 1%, respectively) of all knee arthroplasty procedures performed, whereas the combined rate of isolated medial and lateral disease is 30% to 40%. This discrepancy may be attributed to hesitancy associated with a lack of familiarity with the procedure or failure to recognize isolated compartment disease. Furthermore, the 10:1 ratio of medial to lateral UKA could also be attributed to a lack of familiarity with the procedure and the increased difficulty of lateral UKA because of the screw-home mechanism, which complicates the kinematic profile of the lateral compartment.[5]

There are a limited number of studies investigating the survival of lateral UKA when compared with medial UKA, but the most recent data suggest that lateral UKA can be just as effective of a procedure as the medial UKA.[5] Outcomes hinge on proper patient and implant selection and surgical technique.

INDICATIONS

Patients that are being considered for lateral UKA should have isolated lateral compartment disease radiographically and by examination. Berend and colleagues[5] also argue that minor patellofemoral disease may also be ignored. In addition to isolated lateral compartment disease, varus and valgus stress radiographs demonstrating a correctable deformity with maintenance of the medial joint space are usually adequate for identifying isolated lateral disease. Argenson and colleagues[6] showed improved long-term survivorship after adopting the practice of evaluating opposite femorotibial compartment and the flexibility of the deformity using stress radiographs.

CONTRAINDICATIONS

Patients with significant disease in more than one compartment, a fixed valgus deformity, ligamentous deficiency, less than 90 degrees of flexion, or inflammatory arthritis should not be considered for this procedure.

SURGICAL TECHNIQUE OF LATERAL UNICONDYLAR KNEE ARTHROPLASTY

The senior author uses an extramedullary tibial guide and an extramedullary femoral guide following implant techniques according to the implant manufacturer's technique guideline.[7] The components include a spherical femoral component with a nonmodular, metal-backed, fixed-bearing tibial design. A fixed-bearing device for lateral UKA is recommended because of the high range of motion, femoral posterior subluxation, screw-home mechanism, and significant laxity of the lateral compartment in flexion. A summary of the surgical technique used at our institution is described next.

POSITIONING

The patient is placed supine on a standard operating table with a tourniquet placed on the proximal thigh. The operative leg is placed in a hanging leg position with a leg holder on the side of the bed. This leg holder is positioned so the hip is flexed 30 degrees and 135 degrees of knee flexion without impingement on the side of the bed (**Fig. 1**). The nonoperative leg is placed in a padded leg holder, and the foot of the bed is dropped perpendicular to the floor. The leg is then prepared and draped.

APPROACH AND EXPOSURE

An abbreviated midline incision is created from approximately 2 cm proximal to the superior pole of the patella, extending to the proximal, lateral aspect of the tibial tubercle. Through this incision, a lateral parapatellar approach is performed with careful dissection of the superficial fascia and preservation of the infrapatellar fat pad. Lateral tibial and femoral osteophytes are excised. The visible part of the lateral meniscus is excised. The front of the tibia, from the tibial tubercle to the rim of the plateau and Gerdy tubercle, is exposed. Isolated lateral disease and an intact anterior cruciate ligament are confirmed before proceeding.

TIBIAL CUT

An extramedullary tibial guide is placed to set the varus/valgus alignment and slope. The amount of slope depends on manufacturers' recommendations and for this system is set at 0 degrees.

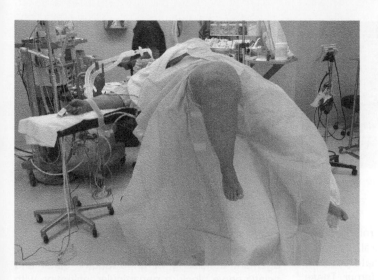

Fig. 1. Leg holder is positioned so the hip is flexed 30 degrees and 135 degrees of knee flexion without impingement on the side of the bed.

The patellar tendon is split in line with its fibers (**Fig. 2**). The vertical tibial cut is the first cut made using a reciprocating saw with a stiff narrow blade. This cut should be in line with the medial border of the lateral femoral condyle and internally rotated 10 to 15 degrees from the mid-sagittal plane of the tibia (**Fig. 3**).[8] The transpatellar tendon technique facilitates the proper amount of internal rotation of the tibial component. This allows the femoral component to articulate with the tibial polyethylene evenly throughout the screw-home mechanism and enlarges the surface area of the resection/implant to prevent subsidence.

An Army-Navy type retractor is placed to protect the patellar tendon and the horizontal tibial cut is made using a 12-mm-wide oscillating saw blade (**Fig. 4**). Enough bone must be resected to fit the tibial template and a 5-mm spacer in the flexion gap. A broad osteotome is used to lever up the resected plateau and it is excised along with the remaining soft tissue attachments posteriorly.

This resected bone is matched up against the tibial baseplate trials for sizing (**Fig. 5**).

POSTERIOR CONDYLE RESECTION AND MILLING

An extramedullary guide is used to align the femoral resections. It is aligned parallel to the anatomic axis of the femur. A tibial template is placed, the femoral drill guide is inserted, and a 4-mm spacer in between them. The drill guide ultimately sets the position of the femoral component and should be set parallel to the extramedullary guide in the axial and sagittal plane (**Fig. 6**). A common mistake is to internally rotate the drill guide. This leads to a malpositioned femoral component resulting in impingement on the tibial spine eminence in knee extension through the screw-home mechanism. Placing the drill guide too medial similarly leads to impingement against the tibial spine eminence in extension and edge loading of the tibial polyethylene. To avoid this,

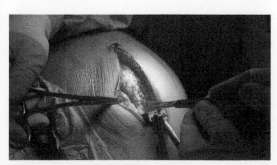

Fig. 2. The patellar tendon is split in line with its fibers.

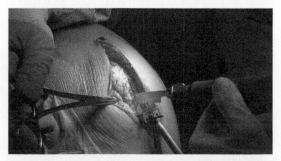

Fig. 3. The vertical tibial cut is made with the medial border of the lateral femoral condyle and internally rotated 10 to 15 degrees from the mid-sagittal plane of the tibia.

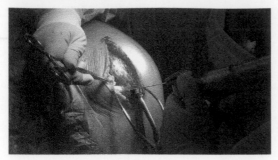

Fig. 4. The horizontal tibial cut is made using a 12-mm-wide oscillating saw blade.

the drill guide should be placed in the middle of the condyle or even cheated slightly lateral.

With the drill guide in the appropriate position, two drill holes are made in the distal femur. These holes are used to make the posterior femur and distal femur resections. A femoral saw block is placed and the posterior femoral resection is made using a broad sagittal saw (**Fig. 7**). This is a measured resection specific to the implant. Balancing is accomplished with milling of the distal femur.

The block is removed and a spigot is placed into the large distal femoral drill hole. The distal femur is prepared by milling over the spigot (**Fig. 8**). Sequential milling is done until the same size spacer block fits comfortably in flexion and extension.

BALANCING THE FLEXION AND EXTENSION GAPS

The flexion and extension gaps are tested with the trials in place. Balancing the gaps differs from a medial unicompartmental or TKA. In the lateral compartment of a normal knee, the flexion gap is loose compared with the extension gap. This normal disparity should be recreated without over-correction. Our preference is to balance 2 to 3 mm lax at 90 degrees of flexion and "tight" or 0 mm at full extension.

INSERTING AND CEMENTING THE FINAL COMPONENT

Multiple small drill holes roughen the femoral and tibial surfaces to improve cement interdigitation. Femoral and tibial components are cemented into place at 45 degrees of flexion (**Fig. 9**). A hemovac drain is placed. The capsular tissue is approximated with #2 Quill PDO, subcutaneous tissue with 0 Quill Monoderm, and the skin is closed with 2–0 Quill Monoderm and Dermabond.

POSTOPERATIVE CARE

Patients are allowed to be weight bearing as tolerated. They are discharged either the day of surgery or on postoperative day 1. Perioperative pain management consisting of an adductor canal and sciatic nerve block, a periarticular infiltration with 20 mL of Exparel (Pacira Pharmaceuticals Inc, Parsipanny, NJ) 1.3%, 25 mL of bupivacaine 0.5%, 0.5 mL of epinephrine 1:1000, and 30 mg of ketorolac, and oral pain medication allows for an accelerated recovery time. Venous thromboembolism prophylaxis is carried out using risk stratification performed by the medical internist. Patients at a lower risk are placed on 325 mg of aspirin twice daily for 6 weeks with sequential compression devices. Those patients determined to be at high risk are usually placed on low-molecular-weight heparin. First postoperative appointment is at 6 weeks for clinical and radiographic examination.

RESULTS OF LATERAL UNICONDYLAR KNEE ARTHROPLASTY
Survivorship in Early Studies

Unicompartmental knee arthroplasty of the medial and lateral compartment has been performed for more than 40 years. Since they were first implanted there have been few studies focused specifically on lateral UKA. Several early studies showed relatively high failure rates largely caused by patient selection criteria, surgical technique, and implant design.

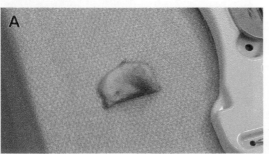
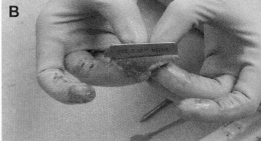

Fig. 5. The resected lateral tibial plateau is matched up against the tibial baseplate trials for sizing.

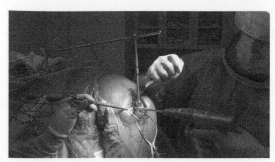

Fig. 6. The drill guide is set parallel to the extramedullary guide.

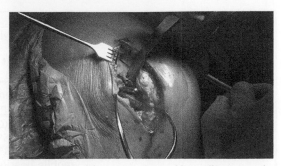

Fig. 8. The distal femur is prepared by milling over the spigot.

Scott and Santore[9] in 1981 reported 83% survivorship on 12 lateral UKAs at 3.5 years. Cameron and colleagues[10] at the same time reported 9 of 20 lateral UKAs achieved poor results. Argenson and colleagues[6] reported an 84% survivorship at 16 years, with four out of five revisions occurring before 1989 when they began evaluating the medial compartment and correction of the deformity with stress radiographs. Failures in all three articles were linked to patient selection criteria, which was not as refined or rigorous as current criteria. Most surgeons now consider a severe or uncorrectable valgus preoperative deformity or advanced degenerative changes of the medial compartment a contraindication to performing a lateral UKA.

The impact of implant design and surgical technique on survivorship is shown in the early experiences of Ashraf and colleagues,[11] Argenson and colleagues,[6] and Gunther and colleagues.[12] Ashraf and colleagues[11] reported on 4 of 15 revision surgeries for the treatment of a fractured femoral component. These all occurred before 1988, when the implant design was modified to incorporate a stronger femoral component. Argenson and colleagues[6] reported one of five revision surgeries was caused by early tibial implant migration. This occurred in a patient operated on early in the study, when limited instrumentation

was available, and cuts were handmade based on a resurfacing concept. The failure was attributed to a technical error secondary to limited instrumentation. Lastly, Gunther and colleagues[12] reported a 21% failure rate using the mobile-bearing Oxford unicompartmental prosthesis in the lateral compartment with a 10% rate of bearing dislocation. This prosthesis has since been modified to a domed tibial component with a biconcave mobile-bearing polyethylene insert. The new design more closely matches the anatomy of the convex lateral compartment and more closely reproduces normal knee kinematics. This has drastically improved, but not eliminated, the dislocation issue.[13–16]

Modern Results

With modifications in patient selection criteria, surgical technique, and implant design contemporary literature has shown 10-year survivorships well over 90%. See **Table 1** for a review of published results of lateral UKA. Xing and colleagues[17] reported no revisions at 4.5 years in a group of 31 lateral UKAs, as did Sah and Scott[18] at 5 years in a group of 49 knees, and Pennington and colleagues[8] at 12 years in a group of 29 knees.

In two of the largest series, Berend and colleagues[5] reported 99% survivorship in 100 lateral UKA at 3 years and Smith and colleagues[19] showed implant survival for 101 lateral UKA to be

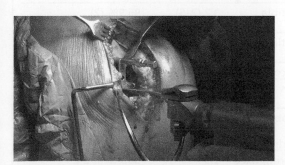

Fig. 7. A femoral saw block is placed and the posterior femoral resection is made using a broad sagittal saw.

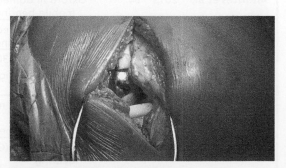

Fig. 9. Final components in place.

Table 1
A review of published results of lateral unicondylar knee arthroplasty

Authors, Year	Number of Knees	Type of Implant (Manufacturer)	Follow-Up (y)	Survivorship (Number of Revisions)
Keblish & Briard,[20] 2004	19	LCS (DePuy), cemented, mobile-bearing	11 (5–19)	84.2% at 11 y (3)
Saxler et al,[21] 2004	46	AMC Uniglide (Corin), 72% cemented, 25% cementless, 3% hybrid, mobile-bearing	5.5 (2.3–12.5)	89% at 5.5 y (5)
O'Rourke et al,[22] 2005	14	Marmor (Smith & Nephew), cemented all-poly tibia	24 (17–28)	72% at 25 y (2)
Pennington et al,[8] 2006	29	Miller-Galante (Zimmer), cemented, metal-backed (75%); all-poly tibia (25%)	12.4 (3.1–15.6)	100% at 12.4 y (0)
Cartier et al,[23] 2007	30	<Age 60, Genesis (Smith & Nephew); 20% cementless; 43% all-poly	(5–14)	94% at 10 y 92% at 11 y 88% at 12 y
Forster et al,[24] 2007	30	Preservation (DePuy), cemented, 13 mobile-bearing; 17 all-poly fixed	2	Mobile: 77% at 2 y (3) Fixed: 100% at 2 y (0)
Sah & Scott,[18] 2007	49	4 different designs	5.2 (2–14)	100% at 5.4 y (0)
Argenson et al,[6] 2008	38	4 different designs	12.6 (3–23)	84% at 16 y (5)
Bertani et al,[25] 2008	35	4 different designs	9 (2–22)	85.7% at 9 y (5)
Lustig et al,[26] 2009	60	HLS Evolution (Tornier), cemented, all-poly tibia	5.2 (2.1–13.3)	98.3% at 5 y; 98.3% at 10 y (11/144)
John et al,[27] 2011	9	Miller-Galante (Zimmer), cemented, metal-backed, fixed-bearing	10.8 (2–16)	97% at 5 y, 41% at 8 y
Pandit et al,[16] 2010	53 65 101	Oxford I & II (Biomet) Oxford III flat tibia Oxford III domed tibia	5.2 4.7 (3–9) 2.3 (1–4)	82% at 4 y (11) 91% at 4 y (9) 98% at 4 y (1)
Berend et al,[5] 2012	100	Vanguard M (Biomet), cemented, metal-backed	3.3 (2–7)	99% (1)
Heyse et al,[28] 2012	50	Genesis (Smith & Nephew), 20 uncemented, 23 all-poly	10.8 (5–16)	94% (3)
Lusting et al,[29] 2012	13	3 different designs	10.2 (3–22)	92.3% (1)
Panni et al,[30] 2012	9	Zimmer High Flex (Zimmer)	4.5 (3–6)	100% (0)
Xing et al,[17] 2012	31	Preservation (Depuy)	4.5 (2–6)	100% (0)
Schelfaut et al,[14] 2013	25	Oxford III domed tibia (Biomet), mobile-bearing	Min 1	96% (1)
Altuntas et al,[13] 2013	64	Oxford III domed tibia, mobile-bearing	3.2 (2–5)	96.9% (2)
Streit et al,[15] 2012	50	Oxford III domed tibia, mobile-bearing	3 (2–4)	94% (3)
Sebilo et al,[31] 2013	82	Implants from 30 companies	5.2 (<1–23)	84% at 10 y
Thompson et al,[32] 2013	30	4 different designs	2	96.4%
Marson et al,[33] 2014	15 12	Oxford domed mobile-bearing Zimmer fixed-bearing	2.9 (1–4) 2.7 (1–6)	93.3% (1) 100% (0)
Smith et al,[19] 2014	101	AMC Uniglide (Corin), fixed-bearing	3.9	98.7% at 2 y 95.5% at 5 y (4)

95.5% at 5 years. Our practice has experienced favorable results consistent with the recent literature.

A retrospective review performed from June 2005 through September 2010 revealed 98 consecutive patients (104 knees) treated with lateral UKA by a single surgeon (KRB). Indications were complete lateral bone-on-bone arthrosis with a correctible deformity and maintenance of the medial joint space on varus stress radiographs. Two knees were posttraumatic; all others were osteoarthritic. A nonmodular, fixed-bearing, metal-backed tibial component was used and all components were cemented. No knee required intraoperative conversion to TKA. A lateral parapatellar approach was used in all cases. There was a preponderance of women (69%). Age averaged 57 years and body mass index averaged 30.0 kg/m^2. Follow-up averaged 28 months (6 weeks–6.2 years). Average Knee Society pain, clinical, and function scores improved from 10.0, 48.8, and 53.3 preoperatively to 41.6, 89.6, and 73.6 at most recent follow-up. Two complications required reoperation: one non-healing wound was treated with incision and debridement and one medial meniscus tear was repaired arthroscopically. One knee required revision to cruciate-retaining TKA at 16 months secondary to loosening of the femoral component and one lateral UKA was revised for pain at an outside institution. Thus, at 2 years average follow-up survival seems to be good.

SUMMARY

Unicompartmental osteoarthritis of the knee is a relatively common disease that is seen in 40% of the population. Although isolated lateral compartment disease is not seen as often as isolated medial compartment disease, it exists with relative frequency and may be treated successfully with UKA. With proper patient selection, surgical technique, and implant choice, early survivorship ranges from 95% to 99%.

REFERENCES

1. Felson DT, Naimark A, Anderson J, et al. The prevalence of knee osteoarthritis in the elderly. The Framingham Osteoarthritis Study. Arthritis Rheum 1987;30(8):914–8.
2. Leyland KM, Hart DJ, Javaid MK, et al. The natural history of radiographic knee osteoarthritis: a fourteen-year population-based cohort study. Arthritis Rheum 2012;64(7):2243–51.
3. Murphy L, Helmick CG. The impact of osteoarthritis in the United States: a population-health perspective: a population-based review of the fourth most common cause of hospitalization in U.S. adults. Am J Nurs 2012;112(3 Suppl 1):S13–9.
4. Kurtz S, Ong K, Lau E, et al. Projections of primary and revision hip and knee arthroplasty in the United States from 2005 to 2030. J Bone Joint Surg Am 2007;89(4):780–5.
5. Berend KR, Kolczun MC II, George JW Jr, et al. Lateral unicompartmental knee arthroplasty through a lateral parapatellar approach has high early survivorship. Clin Orthop Relat Res 2012;470(1):77–83.
6. Argenson JN, Parratte S, Bertani A, et al. Long-term results with a lateral unicondylar replacement. Clin Orthop Relat Res 2008;466(11):2686–93.
7. Biomet, Inc. Vanguard M Partial Knee: lateral and medial surgical technique. Available at: www.biomet. com/orthopedics/getFile.cfm?id=2464&rt=inline.
8. Pennington DW, Swienckowski JJ, Lutes WB, et al. Lateral unicompartmental knee arthroplasty: survivorship and technical considerations at an average follow-up of 12.4 years. J Arthroplasty 2006;21(1):13–7.
9. Scott RD, Santore RF. Unicondylar unicompartmental replacement for osteoarthritis of the knee. J Bone Joint Surg Am 1981;63(4):536–44.
10. Cameron HU, Hunter GA, Welsh RP, et al. Unicompartmental knee replacement. Clin Orthop Relat Res 1981;(160):109–13.
11. Ashraf T, Newman JH, Evans RL, et al. Lateral unicompartmental knee replacement survivorship and clinical experience over 21 years. J Bone Joint Surg Br 2002;84(8):1126–30.
12. Gunther TV, Murray DW, Miller R, et al. Lateral unicompartmental arthroplasty with the Oxford meniscal knee. Knee 1996;3:33–9.
13. Altuntas AO, Alsop H, Cobb JP. Early results of a domed tibia, mobile bearing lateral unicompartmental knee arthroplasty from an independent centre. Knee 2013;20(6):466–70.
14. Schelfaut S, Beckers L, Verdonk P, et al. The risk of bearing dislocation in lateral unicompartmental knee arthroplasty using a mobile biconcave design. Knee Surg Sports Traumatol Arthrosc 2013;21(11): 2487–94.
15. Streit MR, Walker T, Bruckner T, et al. Mobile-bearing lateral unicompartmental knee replacement with the Oxford domed tibial component: an independent series. J Bone Joint Surg Br 2012;94(10):1356–61.
16. Pandit H, Jenkins C, Beard DJ, et al. Mobile bearing dislocation in lateral unicompartmental knee replacement. Knee 2010;17(6):392–7.
17. Xing Z, Katz J, Jiranek W. Unicompartmental knee arthroplasty: factors influencing the outcome. J Knee Surg 2012;25(5):369–73.
18. Sah AP, Scott RD. Lateral unicompartmental knee arthroplasty through a medial approach. J Bone Joint Surg Am 2007;89(9):1948–54.
19. Smith JR, Robinson JR, Porteous AJ, et al. Fixed bearing lateral unicompartmental knee

arthroplasty-short to midterm survivorship and knee scores for 101 prostheses. Knee 2014;21:843–7.

20. Keblish PA, Briard JL. Mobile-bearing unicompartmental knee arthroplasty: a 2-center study with an 11-year (mean) follow-up. J Arthroplasty 2004;19(7 Suppl 2):87–94.

21. Saxler G, Temmen D, Bontemps G. Medium-term results of the AMC-unicompartmental knee arthroplasty. Knee 2004;11(5):349–55.

22. O'Rourke MR, Gardner JJ, Callaghan JJ, et al. The John Insall Award: unicompartmental knee replacement. A minimum twentyone-year followup, end-result study. Clin Orthop Relat Res 2005;440:27–37.

23. Cartier P, Khefacha A, Sanouiller JL, et al. Unicondylar knee arthroplasty in middle-aged patients: a minimum 5-year followup. Orthopedics 2007;30(8 Suppl):62–5.

24. Forster MC, Bauze AJ, Keene GC. Lateral unicompartmental knee replacement: fixed or mobile bearing? Knee Surg Sports Traumatol Arthrosc 2007;15(9):1107–11.

25. Bertani A, Flecher X, Parratte S, et al. Unicompartmental-knee arthroplasty for treatment of lateral gonarthrosis: about 30 cases: midterm results. Rev Chir Orthop Reparatrice Appar Mot 2008;94(8):763–70.

26. Lustig S, Paillot JL, Servien E, et al. Cemented all polyethylene tibial insert unicompartmental knee arthroplasty: a long term follow-up study. Orthop Traumatol Surg Res 2009;95(1):12–21.

27. John J, Mauffrey C, May P. Unicompartmental knee replacements with Miller-Galante prosthesis: two to 16-year follow-up of a single surgeon series. Int Orthop 2011;35(4):507–13.

28. Heyse TJ, Khefacha A, Peersman G, et al. Survivorship of UKA in the middle-aged. Knee 2012;19: 585–91.

29. Lusting S, Parratte S, Magnussen RA, et al. Lateral unicompartmental knee arthroplasty relieves pain and improves function in posttraumatic osteoarthritis. Clin Orthop Relat Res 2012;470:69–76.

30. Panni AS, Vasso M, Cerciello S, et al. Unicompartmental knee replacement provides early clinical and functional improvement stabilizing over time. Knee Surg Sports Traumatol Arthrosc 2012;20: 579–85.

31. Sebilo A, Casin C, Lebel B, et al. Clinical and technical factors influencing outcomes of unicompartmental knee arthroplasty: retrospective multicentre study of 944 knees. Orthop Traumatol Surg Res 2013;99(4 Suppl):S227–34.

32. Thompson SA, Liabaud B, Nellans KW, et al. Factors associate with poor outcomes following unicompartmental knee arthroplasty. J Arthroplasty 2013;28: 1561–4.

33. Marson B, Prasad N, Jenkins R, et al. Lateral unicompartmental knee replacements: early results from a district general hospital. Eur J Orthop Surg Traumatol 2014;24(6):987–91.

Modes of Failure in Metal-on-Metal Total Hip Arthroplasty

Keith A. Fehring, MD[a],*, Thomas K. Fehring, MD[b]

KEYWORDS

- Total hip arthroplasty • Metal-on-metal • Adverse tissue reactions • Corrosion • Cobalt-chromium

KEY POINTS

- When evaluating any patient with a painful total hip arthroplasty, a systematic approach is mandatory regardless of bearing type.
- In metal-on-metal hips, bearing malfunction can occur without the presence of symptoms.
- Metal corrosion and adverse local tissue reaction may occur because of problems with the articulation or any modular junction of the implant.
- Ion levels and cross-sectional imaging techniques (MRI, ultrasound) are beneficial in evaluating a metal-on-metal THA.
- Stratifying the MoM patient into low, moderate, or high risk can help the diagnostic and treatment algorithm.

INTRODUCTION: NATURE OF THE PROBLEM

Metal-on-metal (MoM) total hip arthroplasty (THA) made a resurgence because of its improved wear characteristics, promise of longevity, and lower dislocation rates in the early 2000s.[1,2] By 2006, 35% of primary THA in the United States were MoM articulations. It was estimated that more than 1,000,000 MoM articulations had been implanted worldwide since 1996.[3] Recently, adverse local tissue reactions (ALTRs) associated with these bearings has curbed enthusiasm for their use. New modes of failure associated with these bearings have been identified, in addition to the traditional failure mechanisms.

The evaluation of a failed MoM THA must begin systematically, and should be similar to the evaluation of any problematic THA. Traditional modes of failures, such as instability, infection, tendinitis, aseptic loosening, periprosthetic fracture, and referred pain, must be thoroughly evaluated as potential causes of pain before attributing the source of the problem to the metal bearing.[2,4,5] Once these issues have been ruled out, bearing-related problems, such as tissue necrosis, modular junction corrosion, skin hypersensitivity, and systematic cobaltism, should also be considered.

Histologically ALTRs appear as a lymphocytic inflammatory response that leads to vasculitis-induced necrosis of soft tissue and bone. The terms aseptic lymphocytic vasculitis-associated lesions (ALVAL), pseudotumor, and metallosis have all been used as umbrella terms in the literature to describe the soft tissue destruction caused by metal-metal junctions and articulations in THA.[1,2,4–10] The more commonly accepted term

Funding Sources: None.
Conflict of Interest: None (Dr K. Fehring); Depuy-Johnson and Johnson, Board of Directors-Knee Society, AAHKS – Research support, consultant and royalties (Dr T. Fehring).
[a] Department of Orthopaedic Surgery, Mayo Clinic, 200 First Street Southwest, Rochester, MN 55905, USA;
[b] Ortho Carolina Hip and Knee Center, 2001 Vail Avenue, Charlotte, NC 28209, USA
* Corresponding author.
E-mail address: kfehring@gmail.com

orthopedic.theclinics.com

for these problems is ALTR. This article presents the evaluation and treatment of modes of failure unique to MoM THA.

EVALUATION OF PAINFUL METAL-ON-METAL TOTAL HIP ARTHROPLASTY: A DIAGNOSTIC ALGORITHM

The evaluation of a painful MoM THA is multifaceted, focusing on history and physical examination, radiography, laboratory values, and cross-sectional imaging. A thorough review of systems must be performed because systemic cobaltism has been reported.[11]

Patient History

A thorough patient history is essential in the evaluation of a patient with painful MoM THA.

- The location, duration, and severity of pain are essential to the evaluation.
- Exacerbating or alleviating factors should be noted.
- Signs or symptoms of infection must be delineated in the history, because this changes the diagnostic and treatment algorithm.
- The skin should be inspected for previous scars, dermal reaction, or signs of infection.
- One must also assess for potential hypersensitivity reactions, because these may manifest as past dermatitis in those patients with metal allergy to nickel jewelry.
- A complete review of systems may also unveil systemic issues caused by metallosis (**Boxes 1** and **2**).

Box 1
Questions to consider in the evaluation of a symptomatic MoM patient

Where is the pain?

How long has the pain occurred?

Was there a pain-free interval?

Is there start-up pain?

Is there thigh pain (stem or socket pain)?

Is there groin pain (socket pain)?

Do they have mechanical symptoms?

Exacerbating activities?

Alleviating activities?

Constitutional symptoms?

Instability events?

Box 2
Questions asked during a review of systems because of multiorgan toxicity of cobalt and chromium

Have you had any change in your vision?

Have you experienced any ringing in your ears, difficulty hearing, or dizziness?

Have you experienced recurrent rashes?

Do you have a tremor, difficulty remembering things, or numbness and tingling in your feet and hands?

Do you have shortness of breath?

Do you have mood swings, fatigue easily, or have gained weight lately?

Physical Examination

Physical examination remains important in the evaluation of any painful THA.

- The skin should be inspected for previous scars, dermal reaction, or signs of infection.
- Palpation should be performed to detect any areas of pain or a soft tissue mass.
- Complete neurovascular examination.
- Range of motion of the hip joint and abductor muscle strength testing should be routinely performed.
- Any gait abnormalities, such as a Trendelenburg gait, should be noted.
- Is the pain reproduced by supine or reverse straight leg raising (radiculopathy)?
- Is the pain reproduced by trochanteric palpation (trochanteric bursitis)?
- Is the pain reproduced by resisted hip flexion (iliopsoas tendonitis)?

Radiographic Evaluation

After a complete history and physical, evaluation of a painful MoM THA should proceed with standard radiographs examining implant type and component position, and signs of loosening or osteolysis. One must pay close attention to component malposition, because this has been shown to correlate with increased ion levels and wear. A high abduction angle leads to diminished bearing lubrication leading to increased ion release and soft tissue reactions.[12–17] Radiographic evaluation of the failed THA should include an anteroposterior view of the pelvis and a cross-table lateral view of the affected hip. Both the acetabular and femoral components should be examined closely for signs of loosening or ingrowth. Judet views may be necessary to evaluate for osteolysis or loosening.

Laboratory Testing

Following initial evaluation, laboratory testing is important in the diagnostic algorithm of the painful MoM THA. Erythrocyte sedimentation rate and C-reactive protein should be obtained to rule out periprosthetic joint infection. Unlike metal-on-polyethylene THA, erythrocyte sedimentation rate and C-reactive protein have been shown to be more nonspecific in the evaluation of MoM THA, because patients with ALTR without infection have also shown elevated markers. Likewise, aspiration results of painful MoM THA can be misleading and must be interpreted with caution. Traditional values of 3000 white blood cells per milliliter combined with greater than 80% polymorphonuclear leukocytes (PMN) indicating periprosthetic infection may not apply to MoM THA with ALTR.[18,19] It is therefore important to have a manual rather than an automated cell count performed because automated counts may misinterpret metallic debris leading to spuriously elevated counts.

Metal ion levels (cobalt and chromium) have been used for the evaluation of MoM THA.[1,8,20] These metal ions are not only released from the bearing surface during articulation, but also from modular junctions because of corrosion. In 2010, the British Medicine and Healthcare Products Regulatory Agency voiced concern about MoM hip implants issuing a safety alert recommending cross-sectional imaging in any MoM hip arthroplasty patient with cobalt or chromium ion levels greater than 7 ppb.[10] Although a useful adjunct, ion levels alone should not be used as a trigger for revision because of their inaccuracy in predicting soft tissue damage in MoM THA. Metal ion levels and their correlation to MoM THA are poorly understood and have been unreliable predictors of soft tissue destruction at the time of revision arthroplasty.[4,10,16] Unfortunately, no current test can predict periarticular necrosis; however, biomarkers to detect ALTRs are currently under investigation (**Box 3**).[4,10]

The evaluation of a MoM patient is similar to the evaluation of a potential periprosthetic infection.

Box 3
Laboratory tests used in the evaluation of a painful MoM Hip Arthroplasty

- C-reactive protein
- Erythrocyte sedimentation rate
- Aspiration
- Cobalt
- Chromium

Whereby the clinician cannot rely solely on a single variable to determine the need for intervention, multiple variables must be considered and taken into account as a group (**Fig. 1**).

Advanced Imaging

Cross-sectional imaging in the form of ultrasound or metal artifact reduction sequence (MARS) MRI has been used in the evaluation of adverse soft tissue reactions.[21,22] Ultrasound has been able to detect soft tissue lesions, and may differentiate these lesions as solid or cystic. However, this imaging modality remains operator dependent limiting its consistent use in the detailed evaluation of soft tissue lesions. It can be efficient and cost-effective as an initial screening test with high sensitivity.[21]

MARS MRI has become the workhorse imaging modality for the evaluation of ALTRs associated with MoM THAs.[21,22] MARS MRI allows for early detection of soft tissue lesions and the ability to follow MoM THA patients longitudinally with serial evaluations (**Fig. 2**).

Clinical Presentation

The clinical presentation of a patient with an ALTR remains variable with each patient having an individualized response to metal debris. The initial presenting symptoms may be pain, mechanical symptoms, abductor weakness, instability, or rash.[4,5]

In addition to symptomatic patients, ALTRs have been identified in asymptomatic patients. A recent investigation has shown a 31% prevalence of cystic ALTRs in asymptomatic MoM patients on MARS MRIs.[7] The natural history of these lesions remains undefined but calls into question the reliability of pain as an indicator of bearing malfunction.

RISK STRATIFICATION

Risk stratification is important in the diagnostic and treatment algorithm of the painful MoM

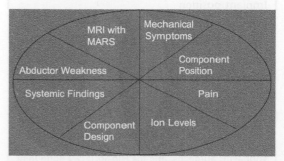

Fig. 1. Important diagnostic MoM variables. MARS, metal artifact reduction sequence.

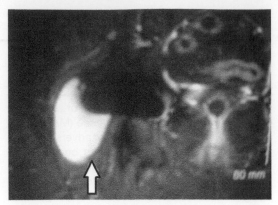

Fig. 2. Cross-sectional MRI of a cystic ALTR lesion (*arrow*) in a MoM THA.

THA. This process is multifactorial because differences in clinical presentation exist. Clinical, laboratory, and radiographic factors help the clinician place patients into low-, moderate-, and high-risk categories, which can affect surveillance and treatment. A patient who is asymptomatic with negative ion levels, appropriately positioned components, and an implant with a low failure rate must be evaluated differently than a patient who is symptomatic with elevated cobalt and chromium levels, a malpositioned cup, and has an implant with a high rate of MoM failures. This risk stratification algorithm has been described by Kwon and colleagues[5] (**Boxes 4–6**).

Box 4
The following factors can help surgeons risk stratify patients

Patient factors

Symptoms

Clinical examination

Implant type

Implant position

Radiographs

Infection work-up

Metal ion level

Cross-sectional Imaging

Data from Kwon YM, Lombardi AV, Jacobs JJ, et al. Risk stratification algorithm for management of patients with metal-on-metal hip arthroplasty: consensus statement of the American Association of Hip and Knee Surgeons, the American Academy of Orthopaedic Surgeons, and the Hip Society. J Bone Joint Surg Am 2014;96(1):e4.

Box 5
Guide to management

Risk stratification can help guide management

Who needs cobalt and chromium levels?

Who needs a MARS MRI?

What frequency of surveillance?

Who needs a revision THA?

METAL-ON-METAL MODES OF FAILURE AND SPECIFIC EVALUATION
Biologic Mechanism of Failure in Metal-on-Metal Total Hip Arthroplasty

The biologic response to metal particle debris can be systemic and local. Much of the concern in THA has been because of the ALTRs caused by the inflammatory response to metal debris. These local responses can result in tissue necrosis and adverse soft tissue reactions. The biologic response to metal particles is not fully understood. It is likely a type IV hypersensitivity response initiating T lymphocytes and macrophages to create a cytotoxic inflammatory response.[1,2,23] Each individualized patient may have a unique response to metal debris. The delayed hypersensitivity reaction driven by T lymphocytes was originally described as ALVAL.[24] Histologically these lesions have an abundance of perivascular lymphocytic reaction leading to vessel constriction and necrosis.

Aseptic Lymphocyte-Dominated Vasculitis-Associated Lesion/Adverse Local Tissue Reactions

The terms ALVAL, ALTR, pseudotumor, and metallosis have all been used as umbrella terms in the literature to describe adverse local soft tissue

---

Box 6
Traditional modes of failure for THA that must also be considered during the evaluation of a MoM THA

Periprosthetic infection

Osteolysis

Aseptic loosening

Dislocation

Periprosthetic fracture

Iliopsoas tendonitis

Referred radicular pain

Trochanteric bursitis

destruction caused by metal debris from MoM articulations and junctions in THA. ALVAL is a histologic term denoting an ALVAL. ALTR, however, is the more accepted term for any ALTR around a MoM THA.

ALTR can be the result of bearing debris or various types of corrosion produced at different MoM articulations within the total hip system. Such corrosion occurs not only at a MoM articulation, but can also be seen because of mechanically assisted crevice corrosion at metal-metal modular junctions, such as the head-neck and neck-stem junctions (**Figs. 3–5**).

Corrosion in Hip Arthroplasty

Modularity in THA offers advantages of intraoperative flexibility to help restore leg length, offset, native biomechanics, and stability. This advantage of modularity does not come without a cost. Corrosion in THA is a newly identified cause of periprosthetic failure.[25–29] Corrosion at the head-neck and neck-body junctions has been linked to modular THA components giving rise to ALTRs. This reaction has been seen in MoM bearings, and metal-on-polyethylene. Taper corrosion can occur between multiple articulations in the THA implant system. There can be MoM articulations at the head-neck junction and the neck-body junction of the femoral component. Multiple types of periarticular corrosion exist. Although galvanic corrosion (corrosion between two dissimilar metals) is well understood, this is not a common failure mode in THA. Alternatively crevice corrosion can occur between modular THA junctions. Mechanically assisted crevice corrosion between two metallic surfaces can wear away the protective oxide layers on the metal surfaces. Once the oxide layer is compromised, corrosion at the junction can occur through a complex chemical

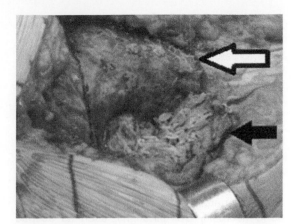

Fig. 4. ALTR seen intraoperatively with necrotic abductor tissue (*white arrow*) and posterior capsule/external rotators (*black arrow*).

reaction. Large areas of corrosion can lead to ALTRs and soft tissue necrosis. Diagnosis can be aided by the measurement of cobalt and chromium ion levels and MARS MRI.

Treatment involves eliminating the cause of the corrosion and limiting the amount of cobalt and chromium in the system. Taper corrosion is often treated with headball exchange with placement of a ceramic headball with a titanium sleeve. If the corrosion is caused by a modular neck interface, revision of the femoral stem may be necessary.

Skin Hypersensitivity

Metal-induced hypersensitivity reactions have been reported at an incidence of 1%.[1] Hypersensitivity following MoM hip arthroplasty seems to be low, but surgeons should be aware of the possibility of this delayed-type lymphocytic response to metal particles when evaluating the symptomatic MoM THA.[23]

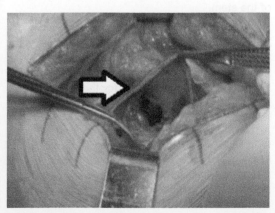

Fig. 3. Capsular metallosis (*arrow*) seen intraoperatively in MoM THA.

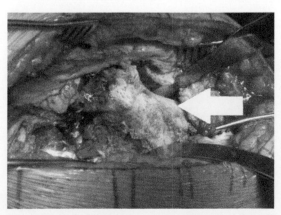

Fig. 5. Abductor deficiency with soft tissue and bone necrosis (*arrow*) from ALTR.

Articulation Modes of Failure

The unique wear characteristics of MoM implants have created problems relating to metal ion release and metallosis. The particles produced by wear of the articulation are more numerous, but smaller in size than the particles produced in metal-on-polyethylene bearings. MoM THAs traditionally have had larger head sizes creating a larger surface area. These designs lead to dissolution of soluble ions, such as cobalt and chromium, increasing their levels in the joint and later the blood. These elevated metal ion levels can initiate an inflammatory cascade leading to tissue and bone necrosis. Complications, such as aseptic loosening and lack of cup ingrowth, have been attributed to equatorial seizing between the cup and large headball.

MoM implants perform best if well lubricated. A high abduction angle leads to diminished bearing lubrication leading to increased ion release and soft tissue reactions.[12–17] A relatively horizontal cup position may increase lubrication leading to improved wear characteristics. Unfortunately, the clinical problems seen with MoM articulations were not predicted by simulator tests. These tests did not account for edge loading that is seen in vivo and thought to be one of the contributing factors to increased wear (**Fig. 6**).[30]

Trunnionosis

Trunnionosis is the phenomenon whereby wear particles are produced at the head-neck junction (trunnion) in modular THA causing corrosion.[31,32] These particles can lead to ALTRs in the surrounding soft tissues. Histologically, these lesions have a classic appearance of a periarticular lymphocytic response similar to that seen in a MoM THA. This type of reaction is not specific to MoM THA and can be seen in metal-on-polyethylene articulations

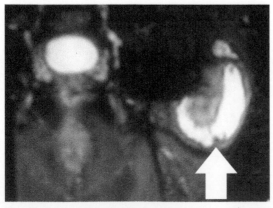

Fig. 6. MARS MRI showing mixed cystic and solid lesion in trochanteric region (*arrow*).

as well if one of the modular components is cobalt chrome.[1,6,29,33,34] It seems to be more prevalent in those patients with larger head sizes. As the size of the head increases, the lever arm on the head-neck taper imparts a significant torque force at this junction causing mechanically assisted crevice corrosion. In this situation, the ion levels are elevated with the cobalt level being higher than the chromium level.[31,32]

If trunnionosis is encountered at the time of revision surgery, the trunnion should be cleaned carefully. If severe corrosion is not present, stem retention is usually preferred because of the morbidity encountered with removal of well-fixed cementless stem. Revision consists of eliminating as much of the cobalt from the system as possible, thereby revising the head to a ceramic head with a titanium sleeve. As with MoM bearing revisions, there should be a drop in the cobalt and chromium ion levels after revision.

Modular Neck Metallosis

Modular necks for THA were introduced with the hope of adding more intraoperative flexibility with regards to leg length, offset, and stability. Unfortunately these implant designs have been fraught with problems including fracture, dissociation, the release of metal debris, and corrosive wear at the neck-body junction of these implants.[27,35,36] This corrosion leads to similar ALTRs as seen with MoM THA.[25] It is important for surgeons to understand the problems associated with modular junctions in THA and have a heightened sense of suspicion for adverse tissue reactions caused by corrosion in these implants.

The treatment of metal corrosion caused by a modular neck implant needs to be individualized depending on a patient's comorbidities, but usually requires femoral revision.[27] Manufacturer-specific tools may be available to facilitate removal of the stem.

Metallosis After Hip Resurfacing

Hip resurfacing grew in popularity because of its bone-preserving nature, and prospects of improved wear and stability for the young, active patient. Hip resurfacing implant designs have also shown a propensity for wear-related issues and ALTRs.[14,15,37] Because there are no modular junctions in the system, ALTRs and ion levels may seem less severe than in monoblock MoM THAs. A 3.1% rate of metallosis at 5 years has been previously reported.[38] The release of metal wear debris at the articulation can also initiate a cascade of inflammatory responses resulting in ALTRs similar to other MoM designs. Radiographic signs of impingement should be noted and present as indentations in the femoral neck that can lead to neck fracture necessitating revision.[2,39] When evaluating a symptomatic patient with a hip resurfacing, the surgeon should have a low threshold for obtaining ion levels and cross-sectional imaging.

Systemic Cobaltism

Systemic cobaltism has been reported to occur because of periprosthetic metallosis from MoM hip arthroplasty. Systemic symptoms of cobaltism include tinnitus, fatigue, vision disturbances, anxiety, hearing loss, neuropathy, and cardiomyopathy.[11] One author noted extremely high cobalt levels in those patients with impaired renal function.[11] Surgeons should be aware of this rare but serious condition when evaluating a symptomatic MoM THA. Most symptoms resulting from cobaltism resolve after revision surgery.

Results of Treatment

The outcomes of revision surgery for metallosis in MoM hip arthroplasty are suboptimal. Early results of the revision of monoblock MoM THA have shown an unfortunately high complication rate ranging from 20% to 38%.[40–42] The most common complications include instability and aseptic loosening of the revised acetabular component thought to be secondary to soft tissue and bony necrosis.[40–42] An alarming 8.1% rate of infection following revision of failed MoM hip arthroplasty has been reported.[43]

SUMMARY

The evaluation of a symptomatic patient following MoM hip arthroplasty remains challenging. It is important to consider all common modes of failure associated with a conventional THA, in addition to those modes of failure unique to MoM articulations. A thorough clinical evaluation, in addition to specialized testing and imaging, is important to make the proper diagnosis. The early recognition of ALTRs is essential for the successful management of the MoM patient. A systematic approach involving a careful history, physical, and radiographic examination should be undertaken in each MoM patient. Ion levels and cross-sectional imaging are useful adjuncts in determining the need for revision. As in evaluating a patient for periprosthetic infection, isolated variables should not trigger the need for surgical intervention. Rather, multiple clinical and diagnostic variables should be used in making such a decision.

REFERENCES

1. Jacobs JJ, Urban RM, Hallab NJ, et al. Metal-on-metal bearing surfaces. J Am Acad Orthop Surg 2009;17(2):69–76.
2. Browne JA, Bechtold CD, Berry DJ, et al. Failed metal-on-metal hip arthroplasties: a spectrum of clinical presentations and operative findings. Clin Orthop Relat Res 2010;468(9):2313–20.
3. Bozic KJ, Kurtz S, Lau E, et al. The epidemiology of bearing surface usage in total hip arthroplasty in the United States. J Bone Joint Surg Am 2009;91(7):1614–20.
4. Kwon YM, Jacobs JJ, MacDonald SJ, et al. Evidence-based understanding of management perils for metal-on-metal hip arthroplasty patients. J Arthroplasty 2012;27(8 Suppl):20–5.
5. Kwon YM, Lombardi AV, Jacobs JJ, et al. Risk stratification algorithm for management of patients with metal-on-metal hip arthroplasty: consensus statement of the American Association of Hip and Knee Surgeons, the American Academy of Orthopaedic Surgeons, and the Hip Society. J Bone Joint Surg Am 2014;96(1):e4.
6. Bisseling P, Tan T, Lu Z, et al. The absence of a metal-on-metal bearing does not preclude the formation of a destructive pseudotumor in the hip: a case report. Acta Orthop 2013;84(4):437–41.
7. Fehring TK, Odum S, Sproul R, et al. High frequency of adverse local tissue reactions in asymptomatic patients with metal-on-metal THA. Clin Orthop Relat Res 2014;472(2):517–22.
8. Engh CA Jr, MacDonald SJ, Sritulanondha S, et al. 2008 John Charnley Award: metal ion levels after metal-on-metal total hip arthroplasty: a randomized trial. Clin Orthop Relat Res 2009;467(1):101–11.
9. Haddad FS, Thakrar RR, Hart AJ, et al. Metal-on-metal bearings: the evidence so far. J Bone Joint Surg Br 2011;93(5):572–9.
10. Kwon YM, Ostlere SJ, McLardy-Smith P, et al. "Asymptomatic" pseudotumors after metal-on-metal hip resurfacing arthroplasty: prevalence and metal ion study. J Arthroplasty 2011;26(4):511–8.
11. Tower SS. Arthroprosthetic cobaltism: neurological and cardiac manifestations in two patients with metal-on-metal arthroplasty: a case report. J Bone Joint Surg Am 2010;92(17):2847–51.
12. Kennedy JG, Rogers WB, Soffe KE, et al. Effect of acetabular component orientation on recurrent dislocation, pelvic osteolysis, polyethylene wear, and component migration. J Arthroplasty 1998;13(5):530–4.
13. Angadji A, Royle M, Collins SN, et al. Influence of cup orientation on the wear performance of metal-on-metal hip replacements. Proc Inst Mech Eng H 2009;223(4):449–57.
14. Langton DJ, Sprowson AP, Mahadeva D, et al. Cup anteversion in hip resurfacing: validation of EBRA

and the presentation of a simple clinical grading system. J Arthroplasty 2010;25(4):607–13.

15. Langton DJ, Joyce TJ, Jameson SS, et al. Adverse reaction to metal debris following hip resurfacing: the influence of component type, orientation and volumetric wear. J Bone Joint Surg Br 2011;93(2):164–71.

16. Hart AJ, Sabah SA, Bandi AS, et al. Sensitivity and specificity of blood cobalt and chromium metal ions for predicting failure of metal-on-metal hip replacement. J Bone Joint Surg Br 2011;93(10):1308–13.

17. Hart AJ, Skinner JA, Henckel J, et al. Insufficient acetabular version increases blood metal ion levels after metal-on-metal hip resurfacing. Clin Orthop Relat Res 2011;469(9):2590–7.

18. Ghanem E, Parvizi J, Burnett RS, et al. Cell count and differential of aspirated fluid in the diagnosis of infection at the site of total knee arthroplasty. J Bone Joint Surg Am 2008;90(8):1637–43.

19. Schinsky MF, Della Valle CJ, Sporer SM, et al. Perioperative testing for joint infection in patients undergoing revision total hip arthroplasty. J Bone Joint Surg Am 2008;90(9):1869–75.

20. MacDonald SJ. Can a safe level for metal ions in patients with metal-on-metal total hip arthroplasties be determined? J Arthroplasty 2004;19(8 Suppl 3):71–7.

21. Garbuz DS, Hargreaves BA, Duncan CP, et al. The John Charnley Award: Diagnostic accuracy of MRI versus ultrasound for detecting pseudotumors in asymptomatic metal-on-metal THA. Clin Orthop Relat Res 2014;472(2):417–23.

22. Potter HG, Nestor BJ, Sofka CM, et al. Magnetic resonance imaging after total hip arthroplasty: evaluation of periprosthetic soft tissue. J Bone Joint Surg Am 2004;86-A(9):1947–54.

23. Willert HG, Buchhorn GH, Fayyazi A, et al. Metal-on-metal bearings and hypersensitivity in patients with artificial hip joints. A clinical and histomorphological study. J Bone Joint Surg Am 2005;87(1):28–36.

24. Watters TS, Cardona DM, Menon KS, et al. Aseptic lymphocyte-dominated vasculitis-associated lesion: a clinicopathologic review of an underrecognized cause of prosthetic failure. Am J Clin Pathol 2010;134(6):886–93.

25. Cooper HJ, Urban RM, Wixson RL, et al. Adverse local tissue reaction arising from corrosion at the femoral neck-body junction in a dual-taper stem with a cobalt-chromium modular neck. J Bone Joint Surg Am 2013;95(10):865–72.

26. Messana J, Adelani M, Goodman SB. Case report: pseudotumor associated with corrosion of a femoral component with a modular neck and a ceramic-on-polyethylene bearing. J Long Term Eff Med Implants 2014;24(1):1–5.

27. Kop AM, Swarts E. Corrosion of a hip stem with a modular neck taper junction: a retrieval study of 16 cases. J Arthroplasty 2009;24(7):1019–23.

28. Hsu AR, Gross CE, Levine BR. Pseudotumor from modular neck corrosion after ceramic-on-polyethylene total hip arthroplasty. Am J Orthop (Belle Mead NJ) 2012;41(9):422–6.

29. Mao X, Tay GH, Godbolt DB, et al. Pseudotumor in a well-fixed metal-on-polyethylene uncemented hip arthroplasty. J Arthroplasty 2012;27(3):493.e13–7.

30. Underwood RJ, Zografos A, Sayles RS, et al. Edge loading in metal-on-metal hips: low clearance is a new risk factor. Proc Inst Mech Eng H 2012;226(3):217–26.

31. Pastides PS, Dodd M, Sarraf KM, et al. Trunnionosis: a pain in the neck. World J Orthop 2013;4(4):161–6.

32. Jacobs JJ, Cooper HJ, Urban RM, et al. What do we know about taper corrosion in total hip arthroplasty? J Arthroplasty 2014;29(4):668–9.

33. Lin KH, Lo NN. Failure of polyethylene in total hip arthroplasty presenting as a pelvic mass. J Arthroplasty 2009;24(7):1144.e13–5.

34. Walsh AJ, Nikolaou VS, Antoniou J. Inflammatory pseudotumor complicating metal-on-highly cross-linked polyethylene total hip arthroplasty. J Arthroplasty 2012;27(2):324.e5–8.

35. Ellman MB, Levine BR. Fracture of the modular femoral neck component in total hip arthroplasty. J Arthroplasty 2013;28(1):196.e1–5.

36. Sotereanos NG, Sauber TJ, Tupis TT. Modular femoral neck fracture after primary total hip arthroplasty. J Arthroplasty 2013;28(1):196.e7–9.

37. Matthies AK, Henckel J, Cro S, et al. Predicting wear and blood metal ion levels in metal-on-metal hip resurfacing. J Orthop Res 2014;32(1):167–74.

38. Ollivere B, Darrah C, Barker T, et al. Early clinical failure of the Birmingham metal-on-metal hip resurfacing is associated with metallosis and soft-tissue necrosis. J Bone Joint Surg Br 2009;91(8):1025–30.

39. Amstutz HC, Campbell PA, Le Duff MJ. Fracture of the neck of the femur after surface arthroplasty of the hip. J Bone Joint Surg Am 2004;86-A(9):1874–7.

40. Huang DC, Tatman P, Mehle S, et al. Cumulative revision rate is higher in metal-on-metal THA than metal-on-polyethylene THA: analysis of survival in a community registry. Clin Orthop Relat Res 2013;471(6):1920–5.

41. Munro JT, Masri BA, Duncan CP, et al. High complication rate after revision of large-head metal-on-metal total hip arthroplasty. Clin Orthop Relat Res 2014;472(2):523–8.

42. Stryker LS, Odum SM, Fehring TK, et al. Revisions of monoblock metal-on-metal THAs have high early complication rates. Clin Orthop Relat Res 2014. [Epub ahead of print].

43. Wyles CC, Van Demark RE 3rd, Sierra RJ, et al. High rate of infection after aseptic revision of failed metal-on-metal total hip arthroplasty. Clin Orthop Relat Res 2014;472(2):509–16.

Trauma

Preface
Trauma

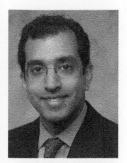

Saqib Rehman, MD
Editor

Fractures of the proximal femur and acetabulum are frequently treated successfully with open reduction internal fixation procedures, but occasionally a patient might end up requiring a total hip arthroplasty. This can be for late posttraumatic arthritis of the hip, or perhaps cutout and failure of primary treatment. In certain cases, it is just better to do the arthroplasty at the initial presentation, especially in elderly patients with dome impaction or acetabular fractures with associated femoral head fractures. This issue of the *Orthopedic Clinics of North America* has two articles dealing with these difficult problems facing orthopedic surgeons who care for these patients. Dr Krause and colleagues have provided an excellent review on total hip arthroplasty after previous fracture surgery. Dr Buller and coauthors have also written an outstanding article entitled, "A Growing Problem: Acetabular Fractures in the Elderly and the Combined Hip Procedure."

Wound management of open fractures, infections, and related problems in orthopedic trauma continues to be critical in both simple and complex fracture management cases. As we all know, nothing ruins a successful fracture reconstruction more than wound breakdown and infection. Dr Gage and colleagues have written an informative article on the uses of negative pressure wound therapy in orthopedic trauma. This continues to be a useful tool in our armamentarium, but many surgeons who only use it occasionally can likely learn a few tips to improve their understanding of when to use it, how to best use it, and when not to use it.

I trust that you will find the trauma section of this issue of the *Orthopedic Clinics of North America* useful to your practice.

Saqib Rehman, MD
Department of Orthopaedic Surgery
Temple University Hospital
3401 North Broad Street
Philadelphia, PA 19140, USA

E-mail address:
Saqib.rehman@tuhs.temple.edu

Orthop Clin N Am 46 (2015) xvii
http://dx.doi.org/10.1016/j.ocl.2014.12.004
0030-5898/15/$ – see front matter © 2015 Published by Elsevier Inc.

Total Hip Arthroplasty After Previous Fracture Surgery

Peter C. Krause, MD*, Jared L. Braud, MD,
John M. Whatley, MD

KEYWORDS

- Total hip arthroplasty • Hip fracture • Posttraumatic arthritis • Failed fracture fixation
- Acetabular fracture • Intertrochanteric fracture • Femoral neck fracture

KEY POINTS

- Total hip arthroplasty can be a very effective salvage treatment for both failed fracture surgery and hip arthritis that may occur after prior fracture surgery.
- The rate of complications is significantly increased including especially infection, dislocation, and loosening.
- Complications are more likely to occur after failed open reduction and internal fixation than after posttraumatic arthritis.
- Adequately ruling out infection before hip arthroplasty can be difficult. The best predictor of infection is a prior infection.
- Long-term outcomes can be comparable to outcomes in other conditions if complications are avoided.

INTRODUCTION

Total hip arthroplasty (THA) is a very effective treatment option for both posttraumatic arthritis that can occur after prior hip fracture surgery and failed hip fracture fixation. Modern acetabular fracture surgery techniques can result in hip preservation and excellent long-term functional outcomes in 70% to 80% of cases.[1,2] Higher-energy fracture patterns, significant articular impaction, and failure to achieve an anatomic reduction can predispose patients to the development of secondary hip arthritis. In patients who are physiologically fit and have failed conservative management, THA can provide appropriate pain control and functional restoration.[3–8]

Avascular necrosis and nonunion after femoral neck fracture surgery, which may occur in 15% to 20% of cases,[9,10] can also be effectively treated with hip replacement.[11] Younger patients with a femoral neck nonunion but with a preserved hip joint can be treated successfully with a valgus intertrochanteric osteotomy.[12] A less common cause of hip posttraumatic arthritis is the femoral head fracture, which may lead to avascular necrosis oftentimes related to an initial traumatic dislocation.

Hip replacement can also be used as a salvage for failed hip fracture surgery.[13–33] If the hip can be saved by revision fixation, it is usually recommended first. Successful functional outcomes with a low rate of complications have been reported

Disclosures: none.
Department of Orthopaedic Surgery, Louisiana State University Health Sciences Center, 1542 Tulane Avenue, 6th Floor, New Orleans, LA 70112, USA
* Corresponding author.
E-mail address: pckrause@mac.com

orthopedic.theclinics.com

with revision internal fixation.[34–36] If the joint is not preserved, then arthroplasty or arthrodesis is the principal surgical option. In cases of older patients with poor bone quality, arthroplasty may be preferable to revision fixation even if the joint is preserved. The published results of THA and hemiarthroplasty in this setting have also been very good with a low rate of serious complications. Rarely, resection arthroplasty should be considered in very ill patients or as a salvage in difficult-to-control infections.

INDICATIONS AND CONTRAINDICATIONS

Patients with significant hip pain with severe arthritis may be candidates for surgery (**Fig. 1**). In the absence of gross implant instability or nonunion, these patients should generally be tried on a nonoperative treatment protocol that includes some combination of antiinflammatories, conditioning, and lifestyle modification before considering surgery. Patients with findings of significant arthritis on radiographs can sometimes function relatively well for years.

In the absence of end-stage arthritis, but in the presence of hardware failure, revision fixation may be an option in otherwise healthy patients. The decision about whether to proceed with revision fixation or hip arthroplasty should be made based on the patient's age and functional status as well as radiographic findings including bone quality. In lower-demand patients, hemiarthroplasty is also an option. Hip fusion is less commonly used now in the younger patient population because of improvements in joint replacement technology. The only absolute surgical contraindication to arthroplasty is an ongoing active infection (**Table 1**).

SURGICAL EVALUATION AND TECHNIQUES AND PROCEDURES
Medical Evaluation

Surgical assessment begins with optimizing the patient medically for surgery. Routine laboratory studies are performed, and patients are seen by their primary care physicians. The authors routinely recommend that patients address

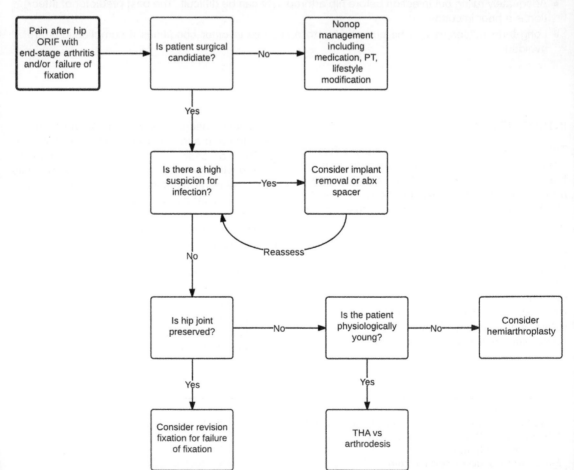

Fig. 1. Decision tree for managing pain after hip fracture surgery.

Table 1 Surgical indications and contraindications	
Indications	**Contraindications**
Posttraumatic hip arthritis	Active infection
Avascular necrosis of the hip	Severe medical comorbidities
Proximal femoral nonunion	Fracture amenable to revision fixation
Loss of fracture fixation	Morbid obesity (BMI >45)

Abbreviation: BMI, body mass index.

Box 1
Preoperative checklist

Dental assessment

Smoking cessation

Local skin issues at the surgical site

Diabetes control

Hold certain medications (eg, plavix, therapeutic monoclonal antibodies for RA, methotrexate)

Weight loss if possible (our usual cutoff for surgery is BMI 40–45)

Abbreviations: BMI, body mass index; RA, rheumatoid arthritis.

---

general health issues as listed in **Box 1** before elective surgery.

Orthopedic Workup

A careful history and physical examination should be performed. Particular attention should be paid to the condition of the abductors (although this is often hard to assess because of pain) and any leg length discrepancy (LLD). A significant leg length difference may be difficult to completely correct at the time of surgery without placing the sciatic nerve at risk.

All patients are carefully screened for infection (**Fig. 2**). If the erythrocyte sedimentation rate and C-reactive protein levels are abnormal or suspicion is prompted by history, examination, or radiographs, a hip aspiration is helpful. Unfortunately, in these cases, unlike revision hip arthroplasty, the presence of a smoldering infection often does not communicate with the joint, making the aspiration less reliable. If an infection is strongly suspected, the decision regarding how to proceed

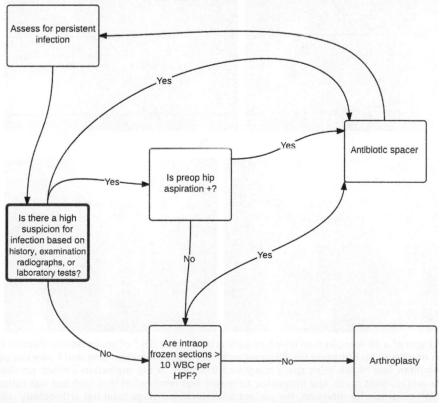

Fig. 2. Decision tree for working up infection before THA. preop, preoperative; WBC per HPF, white blood cells per high power field.

can be made based on frozen section analysis at surgery[7] or the decision in some cases can be made a priori to proceed with a staged reconstruction (**Figs. 3** and **4**). The following aspects of the history should arouse concern:

Any history of infection

Any history of prolonged wound drainage

Any history of repeat surgery for hematoma or seroma

Sudden increase in pain or decline in function and sudden loss of joint space

Extensive periosteal reaction

Periimplant osteolysis

Radiographic Assessment

Bony anatomy should be assessed with pelvic and hip radiographs that show the full extent of the bone that will be instrumented with the planned arthroplasty. The pelvic radiograph is useful in assessing limb length. Oblique radiographs (Judet views) can be useful in defining areas of structural deficiency in the columns and looking for a pelvic discontinuity. Computed tomographic scans are not required but can help in this regard, although frequently scatter from implants degrades the image quality.

Equipment Preparation: Planning for Problems

Every attempt should be made from the radiographs and the medical record to identify exactly what implants are present to facilitate removal. Additional extraction equipment such as a standard broken screw removal set and a metal-cutting high-speed burr should be available at surgery. Appropriate implants should be templated ahead of time, but one should have on-hand bailout implants for possible intraoperative problems

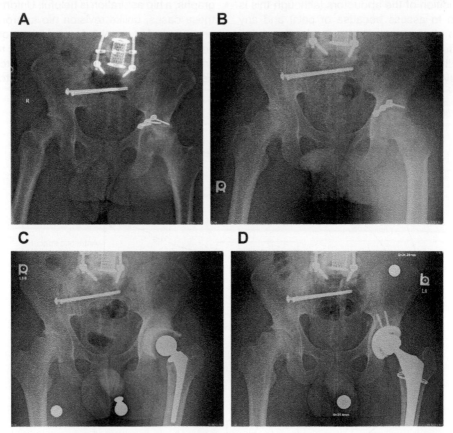

Fig. 3. Radiograph of a 20-year-old man who had early arthritis after ORIF of an acetabular fracture (*A*) and then had a sudden decline in his condition (*B*). Elevated erythrocyte sedimentation rate and C-reactive protein levels and rapid complete loss of the joint space suggested infection. A hip aspiration yielded no fluid, probably because there was no joint space. The intrapelvic hardware was removed at that time but was culture negative. Based on a high suspicion for infection, the patient underwent a 2-stage total hip arthroplasty with an articulated spacer (*C*) followed by a THA (*D*). Operative cultures from the hip debridement showed growth of methicillin-sensitive Staphylococcus aureus (MSSA). Result at 1 year was excellent.

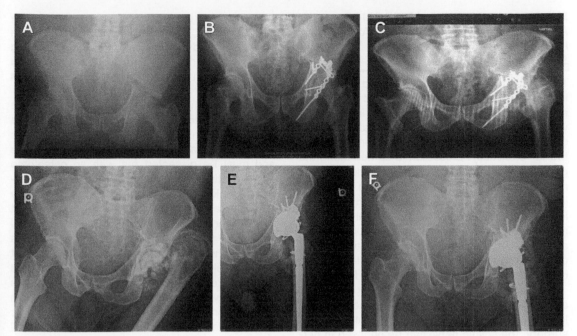

Fig. 4. Radiograph of a 76-year-old man who sustained a transverse posterior wall acetabular fracture (*A*) and had ORIF that was reportedly uncomplicated. Early postoperative radiographs showed arthritis (*B*) that rapidly progressed to joint destruction (*C*). Erythrocyte sedimentation rate and C-reactive protein levels were both elevated. No aspiration was done. Gross pus was present at surgery and the abductors were completely destroyed, so a simple antibiotic cement spacer was placed (*D*) and a 2-stage reconstruction was performed (*E, F*). A satisfactory result was obtained in this low-demand patient, although significant heterotopic ossification is noted.

including periprosthetic femur fracture, acetabular deficiencies including discontinuity, abductor deficiency leading to instability, and operative findings suggesting infection.

Preparation and Patient Positioning

The patient is positioned in the lateral decubitus position on a fully radiolucent operating table with an axillary roll made with a sheet wrapped around a 1-L bag of saline and the down limb padded. The authors prefer to use a peg board but a beanbag positioner may be used. Fluoroscopic imaging should be obtained before the skin preparation to assure proper imaging. Leg lengths should be clinically compared in the supine and lateral position preoperatively because placement in the lateral position will frequently make it appear that the upper leg is shorter than it actually is because of its adducted position. Although clinical judgment of the limb length by palpation in the lateral position is difficult, the authors routinely perform this test as one more way to confirm appropriate length. Skin preparation is with alcohol, followed by a routine chlorhexidine/alcohol combination antiseptic.

Surgical Approach

No single surgical approach can be recommended based on the literature. Most investigators recommend basing the decision about approach on the prior surgical approaches, the existence of heterotopic ossification (HO) or contractures, and the surgeon's preference. The authors' customary approach is the utilitarian posterolateral approach, which is used for virtually all the complex reconstructions that they perform. Through this approach virtually all hardware can be removed and all bony deficits addressed. Rarely intrapelvic hardware needs to be removed via an ilioinguinal or Stoppa approach separately. Other investigators have reported excellent results with the anterolateral approach and the transtrochanteric approach, although, as might be expected, complications with regard to trochanteric fixation have been reported. A digastric osteotomy of the trochanter can be used to extend the surgical approach, which is especially useful after prior intertrochanteric fractures. Regardless of the approach, the published literature suggests that these cases can be exceedingly difficult with reported surgical times of 2 to 6 hours.[17,18,25,28–31]

SURGICAL PROCEDURE: AFTER PRIOR ACETABULAR OPEN REDUCTION AND INTERNAL FIXATION
Step 1: Initial Exposure

The prior scar is incised and extended as needed. If the prior scar is wide and friable, it is routinely excised. The fascia lata is divided in line with the wound being cautious not to denervate a portion of gluteus maximus if the dissection is carried too far proximally. Dissection is carried along the posterolateral aspect of the femur while internally rotating the leg. The capsule is opened at approximately the 1-o'clock position on the left hip, is dislocated, and any remnant femoral head is removed. The piriformis cannot be counted on as a landmark for dissection. If dislocation seems difficult, the femoral neck is cut in situ to avoid causing either a femoral or acetabular fracture.

Heterotopic ossification can block exposure and may need to be removed before the hip is dislocated. Especially after prior acetabular fracture surgery, the sciatic nerve can be encased in heterotopic bone. If the patient has preoperative nerve symptoms, this bone is removed, which can be a tedious procedure. In cases of significant limb length discrepancy or if the nerve is thought to be tethered by scar, the nerve is also dissected out.[37] After dislocating the hip, the head is removed and saved for possible bone graft. If suspicion exists for infection, tissue is sent for frozen section, and routine cultures are done regardless.

Step 2: Exposure and Preparation of the Acetabulum

An anterior Hohmann retractor with a double bend is very useful for retracting the femur anteriorly. This retractor is placed on the anterior wall and the anterior and inferior capsule are excised to facilitate exposure. The exposure of the acetabulum can be extended by subperiosteally dissecting along the anterior and superior acetabulum and by taking down a portion of the gluteus maximus tendon.

Acetabular implants are removed if they impede implant placement, if they are loose, or if there is a suspicion for infection. These plates and screws are almost always completely covered with bone and must be dissected out with an osteotome and sometimes fluoroscopy is helpful. If the implants are left in place, care must be taken not to allow contact with implants that would misdirect the reamer (**Fig. 5**). Removing the most distal screws in a posterior wall plate that extends down to the ischium places the sciatic nerve at considerable risk, and for this reason, the authors try not to remove these plates. On occasion, the authors have used a metal-cutting burr to remove just the portion of the plate blocking exposure or implant placement. Although proximal femoral hardware is usually removed, previous acetabular hardware is frequently left in place if it does not interfere with surgery. The rate of hardware interference has been reported to be from 39% to 81%.[3,6,8]

Care must also be exercised about using local landmarks to judge anteversion of the cup when reaming the acetabulum because the posterior wall is frequently deficient due to the prior injury or can become deficient during hardware removal. Usually the most inferior aspect of the posterior wall is preserved and can help with alignment. Fluoroscopy can be useful for obtaining the correct abduction angle. Reamers can also be misdirected by the sclerotic bone that occurs in prior fracture sites.

A   **B**

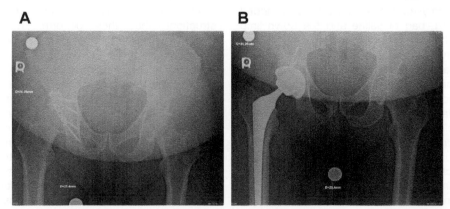

Fig. 5. Radiograph of posttraumatic hip arthritis after ORIF posterior wall fracture 5 years earlier (*A*). During THA most of the implants were removed because the reamer contacted the plate and would have caused eccentric reaming (*B*). The plate was completely encased in heterotopic bone and had to be uncovered from inside out.

Cementless acetabular components have superior results and are routinely used.[3–5] Contained acetabular deficiencies are routinely filled with morselized autograft. Noncontained defects are managed with jumbo cups and metal augments because of the inferior results with structural bone graft. The authors carefully assess for pelvic discontinuity because this must be stabilized at the time of cup placement.

Step 3: Femoral Exposure and Preparation

Femoral preparation after acetabular fracture is usually routine. However, exposure can be more difficult because of stiffness and scar formation. The resection of this scar to enable exposure conversely can result in excessive instability and the natural tendency to overlengthen the extremity. Careful attention to internal landmarks, clinical measurements, and fluoroscopy can help with this. Surgical navigation is also an option.

SURGICAL PROCEDURE: AFTER PRIOR PROXIMAL FEMORAL OPEN REDUCTION AND INTERNAL FIXATION

The initial exposure is complicated by prior fixation hardware and deformity. Appropriate removal equipment including trephines, easy-outs, and metal-cutting burrs need to be available. More difficulty with implant extraction and abductor problems have been reported with cephalomedullary nails than with sliding screw devices or cannulated screws. Care must be taken not to apply excessive torque on the leg to avoid femoral fracture, and consideration should be given to leaving the hardware in place until the hip is dislocated. Exposure can be aided by using the trochanter as a digastric sliding osteotomy leaving the abductors and the vastus lateralis attached.

If the choice is made to proceed with hemiarthroplasty, one then proceeds to femoral exposure and preparation. For THA, reaming of the acetabulum should be undertaken with care because the bone is usually softer than in cases of arthritis and excessive reaming is easily possible.

Most of the literature describes the use of cemented components in these cases, but good results have also been reported with press-fit diaphyseal engaging stems and with the S-ROM stem. Usually, the authors prefer to use a modular stem with diaphyseal fixation in patients with adequate bone stock. If bone quality is good and there is not much deformity, a proximal fit stem may be used (**Fig. 6**). If a cemented stem is used, frequently a calcar replacing component and a long stem is needed. Holes from prior fixation need to be plugged before cementing, which

can easily be done with screws that have been cut with a bolt cutter.[17] If a noncemented stem is used the prior screw holes should be bypassed to avoid a stress riser and a prophylactic cable may be needed.[29] The trochanter is then wired or cabled, but trochanteric fixation problems are common (**Fig. 7**). If the initial fixation device is infected, the case may be managed effectively with a two-stage exchange (**Fig. 8**).

Bercik[38] reported a significantly higher use of diaphyseal fitting implants in patients previously treated with cephalomedullary nails compared to screw and side plate constructs, suggesting that these nails disrupt more proximal metaphyseal bone stock preventing the use of primary metaphyseal press-fit stems. When comparing cannulated screws with screw and side plate constructs for previous femoral neck fractures, Winemaker[21] found no significant difference in blood loss or surgical time. Dehaan[31] also found significantly less operating room (OR) time, implant modularity, and intraoperative transfusions in patients previously treated with cannulated screws compared with those treated either with sliding hip screws or cephalomedullary nails. The sliding hip screw group also trended toward less blood loss, OR time, and implant modularity compared with the nail group, although this did not reach significance. Pui[32] reported a higher complication rate with arthroplasty after cephalomedullary nails than with sliding hip screws including fractures, dislocations, abductor tendon dysfunction, HO, nerve injury, and aseptic loosening.

Previous fracture type also affects intraoperative difficulty in conversion hip arthroplasty. Mortazavi[39] reported a significant difference in the incidence of revision stem use in patients with previous intertrochanteric fractures compared with patients with previous femoral neck fractures. There was also a significantly increased rate of trochanteric osteotomy during surgery for previous intertrochanteric fractures, as well as longer operative time, greater blood loss, and higher transfusion rate. Dehaan found significantly less implant modularity, operative time, and blood loss in previous femoral neck fractures than in peritrochanteric fractures.

Intraoperative fracture is also a concern in these cases. Winemaker reported a higher rate of major (greater trochanter or femoral shaft) fracture complications in the conversion THA group when compared with a matched cohort of patients who underwent primary THA. Dehaan reported an 8.7% rate of intraoperative fracture, all treated successfully with claw plates or cerclage wiring. Zhang reported a 37% greater trochanteric intraoperative

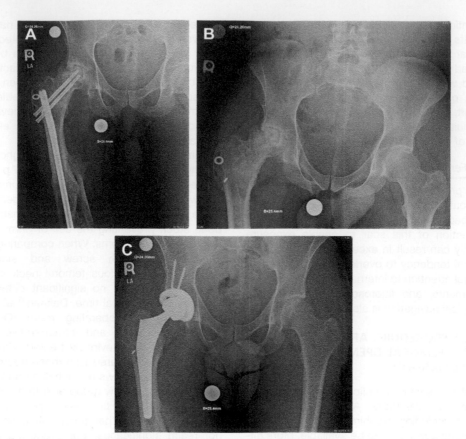

Fig. 6. Radiograph of a 30-year-old man who sustained a segmental femur fracture that was treated with a cephalomedullary nail and went on to avascular necrosis and collapse (A). Infection indices were elevated and therefore the nail was removed initially (B). All cultures gave negative results, and a THA was performed (C). A proximal fit stem was used to avoid the old femoral deformity.

fracture rate, all except one successfully treated with claw plates.[18]

Hip balancing can be especially tricky in these cases, and the hip is likely to have more laxity at the correct length than is typical in arthritis cases. Care should be taken to preserve as much capsule as possible. Larger heads, capsular repair, and anterior approaches reduce the likelihood of dislocation.

COMPLICATIONS AND MANAGEMENT

Complications after conversion THA after previous fracture fixation are, predictably, higher than in cases of primary THA. In the perioperative period, patients have longer surgeries, with greater blood loss and longer hospital stays.[38,39] In the postoperative period, instability, HO, infection, LLD, nerve injury, and loosening have been the major reported complications. Management is primarily by means of awareness and avoidance and prompt management if a complication occurs.

Dislocation

Dislocation is of concern in conversion THA. In the treatment of proximal femur fractures, using a posterior approach, Dehaan[31] reported a 6.5% dislocation rate, with a 4.3% revision rate for recurrent dislocations. A series by Thakur reported no dislocations using a posterior approach; however, a 13% rate of use of a constrained acetabular liners was reported.[29] Zhang reported a 16% dislocation rate, all successfully treated with one closed reduction.[18] Chen reported an 11% rate of dislocation, again treated successfully with closed reduction and abduction bracing.[25] Ranawat[6] reported an overall 9% dislocation rate after previous acetabular fracture, including one patient who underwent a revision surgery for liner exchange because of dislocation. This series, however, did report a 59% use of a lipped liner in the acetabular component.[6] Weber[3] reported 3 total dislocations out of 66 total hip arthroplasties after previous acetabular fracture fixation, with 1 requiring revision because of dislocation. Zhang[8] reported 1

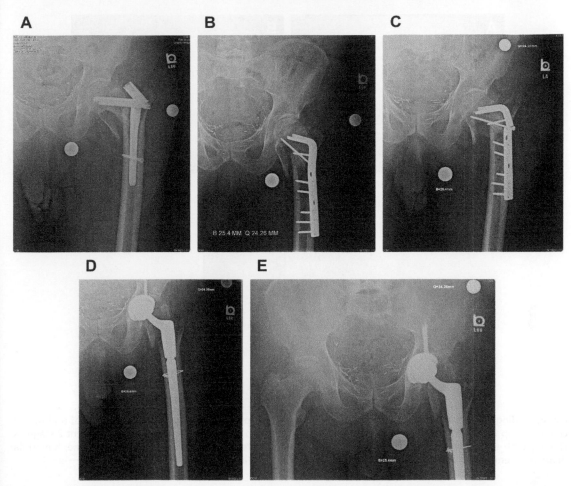

Fig. 7. Radiograph of a 70-year-old man who sustained an unstable intertrochanteric fracture that was treated with a nail and failed (*A*). A revision ORIF was attempted (*B*), but failed (*C*). Although erythrocyte sedimentation rate was elevated, results of cultures were all negative. Therefore a 1-stage THA was performed using press-fit components (*D*, *E*). The soft bone of the pristine acetabulum led to slight overreaming. The tip of the trochanter could not be repaired, but the abductors remained attached distally to preserve function and stability. Functional result was excellent at one year.

dislocation out of 55 hips treated with THA after previous acetabular fracture.

Heterotopic Ossification

HO is always a concern in hip arthroplasty, even more so in the conversion THA population. Dehaan reported a 39% HO rate, with trends toward less HO in patients with previous femoral neck fractures than previous intertrochanteric femoral fractures. Thakur[29] reported a 53% rate of HO; however, the majority was rated at Brooker grade I or II.

Weber[3] reported a low incidence of grade III or IV HO at final follow-up of patients treated with THA after previous acetabular fracture surgery (18% and 2%, respectively) and an overall rate of HO of 58%. Zhang[8] reported 5% grade III HO after

previous acetabular fracture, no grade IV HO, and an overall rate of 29%.

Infection

Infection is also of concern. Dehaan reported a 6.5% deep infection rate, all of which required revision surgery. Chen reported 1 deep infection in a serial debridements of 18, treated successfully with serial debridement and intravenous antibiotics.

In cases of previous acetabular fracture fixation, Ranawat[6] reported infection in 6 of 32 patients, which included 2 patients who had previously been treated nonoperatively for acetabular fracture. Only 2 of these infections were reported as "deep," and 1 death was reported due to complications of deep infection.

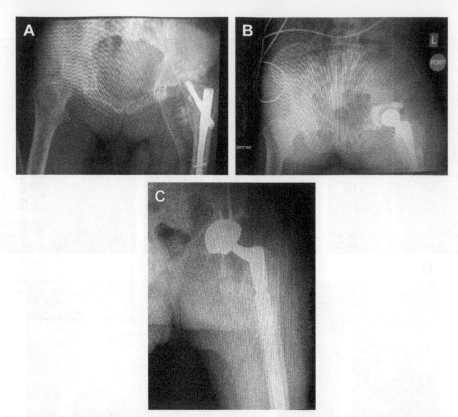

Fig. 8. Radiograph of a 65-year-old man who developed a deep purulent infection after nailing of an intertrochanteric hip fracture and presented with a large draining open anterior wound. (*A*). He underwent 2-stage exchange with an articulated antibiotic spacer with wound closure (*B*). Owing to poor proximal bone, a modular diaphyseal engaging THA was placed at the second stage with a good result (*C*).

Leg-length Discrepancy and Nerve Injury

Thakur[29] reported a mean LLD of 2 mm, ranging from 5 mm shorter to 10 mm longer in conversion hip arthroplasty after previous trochanteric fracture fixation. Weber[3] reported 1 partial peroneal nerve palsy in 66 cases of THA after acetabular fracture fixation. Zhang reported a 5% nerve injury rate in THA after acetabular fracture, of which 1 recovered fully, 1 recovered partially, and 1 failed to show any recovery (**Fig. 9**).

Subsidence and Aseptic Loosening

Chen reported that 2 of 18 patients in his series of diaphyseal fitting press-fit implants had stem subsidence; in both the patients the subsidence stabilized and bony ingrowth was confirmed radiographically. Weber[3] reported 17 revisions due to aseptic loosening in THA after previous acetabular fracture surgery, including 5 loose acetabular components, 7 loose femoral components, and 4 hips with both components loose. There were also 9 additional cases of loosening noted in that series that were not revised, totaling 15 loose

acetabular components and 15 loose femoral components out of 66 total hips. Most of these findings were in the cemented components, and press-fit components may have less loosening.[3–5]

OUTCOMES

Several retrospective reviews have studied THA after operative treatment of fractures about the hip. The outcome data from these articles are difficult to interpret as a whole. The lack of a consistent validated outcome system, the inclusion of a variety of fracture types and treatment failures and the use of several surgical techniques over a long period makes the evaluation difficult. A review of the data is summarized in **Table 2**.

Patients with both operative and nonoperative acetabular fractures go on to hip arthrosis requiring revision or salvage with THA. In Matta's[1,2] initial acetabular fracture case series, 8% (21 of 264) went on to either THA or arthrodesis, and in their later series with longer average follow-up, 15% (124 of 810) underwent conversion. Based on their clinical impression, the investigators concluded that despite the general increased

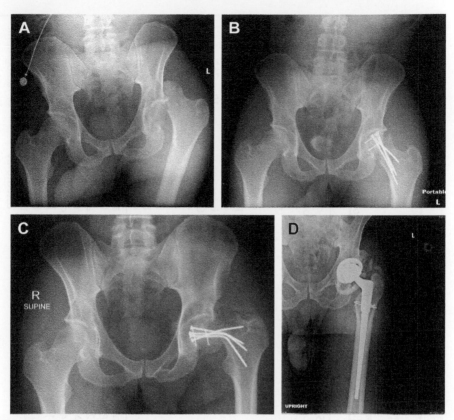

Fig. 9. Radiograph of a 30-year-old man who sustained a femoral head and neck fracture (*A*) that was treated initially with subtoptimal surgical fixation (*B*) and went on to rapid failure (*C*). Infection indices were negative, and a THA was done. An acute lengthening of 3 cm resulted in a delayed-onset foot drop about 4 hours after surgery that resolved with nerve exploration and shortening from a +5 mm head to a −5 mm head. Outcome at 2 years was very good despite Brooker 3 heterotopic ossification (*D*).

difficulty of performing a THA after a failed ORIF of an acetabular fracture, THA can be a reasonably safe, efficacious salvage and can improve the hip function for these patients. Ranawat[6] reviewed a series of 37 THAs for failed acetabular fracture care and found that the average Harris hip score (HHS) increased from 28 to 82 after THA. After revision to THA, the group that had prior surgery had an average HHS of 84 and the group that had been treated nonoperatively had an average of 74. This difference was not statistically significant, so they concluded that outcomes did not differ between operatively and nonoperatively treated acetabular fractures when they have to be revised to THA. Similarly, in 2011, Zhang[8] reported the results of 55 THAs for failed operative or nonoperative treatment of acetabular fractures. The average HHS increased from 49.5 to 90.1. The HHS of the operative group increased from 49.5 to 90.1 and that of the nonoperative fracture care group increased from 54.3 to 92.4. This study also reported no statistical difference between cemented and uncemented THAs.

Bellabarba[4] reported data from a prospective case series of cementless acetabular reconstructions after acetabular fractures; 15 were initially treated with ORIF and 15 were treated nonoperatively. The average HHS increased from 41 to 88 with 90% having good or excellent outcomes. There was 1 revision for aseptic loosening and 4 asymptomatic possibly unstable cups. Radiographically, 67% of the cups had radiolucent lines.

The short-term outcomes for THA for failed ORIF of femoral neck or intertrochanteric femoral fractures when compared with primary THA were reported in 2006 by Winemaker.[21] No difference was found between the 2 groups in HHS, range of motion (ROM), intraoperative complications, postoperative complications, and reoperation rates at 1 year. Global ROM at 1 year was statistically significantly better in the patients treated with cannulated screws at their initial operation when compared with those treated with plate fixation.

When studying only failed ORIF of femoral neck fractures compared with THA done for arthritis, the data differ. Franzen[11] reported on 84 femoral neck

Table 2
Data review: THA after operative treatment of fractures about the hip

Study	Patient # Mean Age	Fracture Type	Treatment	Mean EBL	Mean Operative Time	Complications	Outcomes
Acetabular Fracture							
Weber et al,[3] 1998	66 52 y	Acetabular	THA • 44/66 cementless cups • 46/66 cementless stems	3.5 units transfused	170 min	3 dislocations Loosening • 15 acetabular components • 15 femoral components 1 partial peroneal nerve palsy 0 infections HO • 9/45: grade 0 • 15/45: grade I • 2/45: grade II • 8/45: grade III • 1/45: grade IV	Mean HHS • 49→93 Pain • 4/46 unrevised hips had moderate or severe pain Survival • 10 y: 76% • 15 y: 67%
Bellabarba et al,[4] 2001	30 15 operative 15 nonoperative 51 y	Acetabular	THA for failed acetabular fracture treatment compared with primary THA for OA	Fracture 898 mL 2.2 U transfused OA 413 mL 1.3 U Transfused	179 min 122 min	1 aseptic loosening 4 asymptomatic unstable cups 3 debridements of infected traction pin 1 trochanteric osteotomy nonunion	Mean HHS 41→88 Results • 90% good or excellent Radiolucent lines 67% Survival: revision or radiographic loosening as end point • 10 y: 97%

Study	Patients/Age	Location		Procedure	Blood loss	Complications/Revisions	Clinical follow-up
Berry & Halasy,[5] 2002	34 patients 49.7 y	Acetabular	—	THA: Uncemented acetabular components for failed acetabular fracture treatment	—	9 acetabular revisions • Loosening, dislocation, polywear, or osteolysis; 7 femoral component revisions; 3 minor fractures; 1 dislocation; 1 superficial infection	Clinical follow-up; Pain • 8 no pain • 6 mild pain • 0 patients with moderate or severe pain at final follow-up; Ambulation • 11: unlimited • 1: 6 blocks • 2: <3 blocks
Ranawat et al,[6] 2009	32 24 operative 8 nonoperative 52 y	Acetabular	—	Cementless THA	ORIF 721 mL Nonoperative 711 mL	Dislocation rate 9%; Infection • 6/32	Mean HHS 28→82 • Average HHS ORIF 84 • Average HHS nonoperative 74; Survival • 5 y: 79%
Zhang et al,[8] 2011	55 —	Acetabular	—	THA for failed ORIF or nonoperative acetabular fracture • 47/55 cementless cups • 50/55 cementless stems	—	1 dislocation; 3 sciatic nerve palsy; 3 Brooker III HO; 0 infections	Mean HHS 49.5→90.1 • HHS ORIF 49.5→90.1 • HHS nonoperative 54.3→92.4

(continued on next page)

Table 2
(continued)

Study	Patient # Mean Age	Fracture Type	Treatment	Mean EBL	Mean Operative Time	Complications	Outcomes
Proximal Femur Fracture							
Franzen et al,[11] 1990	84 75 y	Femoral neck	THA Usually posterior approach Cemented	—	—	9/84 failed • 4 permanent dislocation • 2 deep infection • 2 loosening • 1 cup malalignment	Ambulatory status • 11 unaltered • 14 did not use aids • 20 could walk 200 m Age- and sex-adjusted risk for prosthetic failure was 2.5 times after failure of fixation Relative risk of failure by age • <70 y was 1.0 • >70 y was 4.9
Stoffelen et al,[15] 1994	12 79 y	Intertrochanteric and subtrochanteric	4 THA 8 bipolar	—	—	1 dislocation (8.3%) 1 femoral fracture 1 death at 6 wk, due to pneumonia	Merle d'Aubigné hip rating • 45% excellent or very good Ambulation • 18% using ambulator at average 6 mo

Study	N, Age	Fracture Type	Procedure	Blood Loss	OR Time	Complications	Outcomes
Haidukewych & Berry,[17] 2003	60, 78 y	Intertrochanteric	32 THA, 27 bipolar, 1 unipolar	1125 mL	4 h	2 intraoperative fractures with cerclage; 1 hematoma requiring washout; 1 patient with 2 dislocations; 13 medical complications in 12 patients, including 1 death	Pain • 89% no pain or mild pain; Ambulation • 91% able to walk, 59% with 1-arm support or less
Zhang et al,[18] 2004	19, 64.1 y	Intertrochanteric	16 THA, 3 hemiarthroplasty	1378 mL	176 min	7 intraoperative greater trochanteric fractures; 3 dislocations	Mean HHS 38.4→79.8; Ambulation • 50% used cane occasionally or not at all
Winemaker et al,[21] 2006	36, Matched cohort, 71 y	Femoral neck and intertrochanteric	THA	521 mL	95 min	Major complication 13.9% • 4 greater trochanteric fractures • 1 femoral shaft fracture intraoperatively; Major postoperative complications 8.3% • Deep infection with greater trochanteric fracture • Periprosthetic fracture • Superficial infection	Mean HHS 32.5→79.3 at 1 year • HHS not significantly different than matched cohort of primary THA

(continued on next page)

Table 2
(continued)

Study	Patient # Mean Age	Fracture Type	Treatment	Mean EBL	Mean Operative Time	Complications	Outcomes
Laffosse et al,[23] 2007	29 patients 81.1 y	Intertrochanteric	Modular arthroplasty 7 THA 22 bipolar	890 mL	109 min	2 dislocations • 1 requiring revision 2 deaths 2 trochanteric nonunions 0 fractures	Stem subsidence • >5 mm in 3 patients Ambulation • 11 with support • 9 without support • 3 bedridden Pain and function • All reported pain relief and increased function
Lombardi et al,[24] 2007	84 69 y	Femoral neck and intertrochanteric	THA Direct lateral approach	—	—	1 periprosthetic femur fracture 1 HWR for trochanteric plate 1 fascial defect requiring repair 1 washout 0 dislocations	Mean HHS 73.2 Pain score 37.4 Mean lower extremity activity score 7.1
Sharvill et al,[27] 2009	25 73 y	Basicervical femoral neck, intertrochanteric, and reverse oblique	THA	—	—	24% complications • 3 infections • 2 intraoperative fractures • 1 dislocation	Average Oxford hip score 29

Study	N/Age	Fracture	Procedure	Blood Loss	Operative Time	Complications	Outcomes
D'Arrigo et al,[28] 2010	21 75.8 y	Intertrochanteric	19 THA 2 bipolar	—	3 h	Infection • 1 infection requiring explant Fracture • 1 intraoperative femoral fracture treated with cerclage HO • 1 Brooker II at 6 mo	Mean HHS 37 →81 WOMAC • Decreased from 87 preoperatively to 40.8 at 6 mo
Thakur et al,[29] 2011	15 80.6 y	Intertrochanteric	12 THA 3 bipolar	805 mL	183 min	1 DVT 0 dislocation 0 fracture 0 nerve palsy	Mean HHS 35.9→83 Ambulation • 80% walking with cane or less
Abouelela,[30] 2012	16 64 y	12 intertrochanteric 4 subtrochanteric fractures	Modular THA	1068 mL	170 min	8 patients with minor pain 1 greater trochanteric nonunion with 15-mm migration	Mean HHS 17.8→87.7 All Trendelenburg gaits resolved by 6 mo
Bercik et al,[38] 2012	77 hips 74.8 y	Intertrochanteric and femoral neck	THA • Previous screw and side plate or CMN	CMN 700 mL SSP 400 mL	CMN 137 min SSP 113.5 min	—	No HHS Length of stay • No difference

(continued on next page)

Table 2
(continued)

Study	Patient # Mean Age	Fracture Type	Treatment	Mean Operative Time	Mean EBL	Complications	Outcomes
Mortazavi et al,[39] 2012	154 72.8 y	Femoral neck and intertrochanteric	THA Direct lateral approach	Femoral Neck 94 min Intertrochanteric 124 min	Femoral Neck 335 mL Intertrochanteric 659 mL	0 dislocation 21% medical complications after surgery	2.5% required revision surgery
DeHaan et al,[31] 2013	46 64 y	Femoral neck, intertrochanteric, and subtrochanteric	THA Posterior approach	136 min	717 mL	4 fractures 3 deep infections 3 dislocations 1 superficial infection 1 trochanteric bursitis	6 revision • 3 deep infections • 2 recurrent dislocations • 1 aseptic loosening
Pui et al,[32] 2013	91 65 y	Intertrochanteric	THA Posterior, anterolateral	—	—	Significantly higher incidence of complications in CMN compared with SHS	HHS improvements • SHS 41.6→83.6 • CMN 41.6→78.6

Abbreviations: CMN, cephalomedullary nail; DVT, deep venous thrombosis; EBL, estimated blood loss; HHS, Harris hip score; HWR, hardware removal; OA, osteoarthritis; SHS, sliding hip screw; SSP, screw and side plate.

fractures that were salvaged by THA. These arthroplasty results were then compared with those of a cohort of patients with osteoarthritis. Age- and sex-adjusted risk for prosthetic failure was 2.5 times higher after failure of fixation. The relative risk for patients younger than 70 years was 1 but that for patients older than 70 years was 4.9.

Failed intertrochanteric hip fractures can either be treated with revision ORIF or arthroplasty. Haidukewych has reported his experience with both these pathways.[17,36] In a series of 20 revision ORIF performed with bone grafting, 19 of 20 patients showed healing of the fracture and 16 of the 19 who showed healing reported no pain. All patients with healing were ambulatory. However, he noted that these impressive results are in a properly selected population.

For the elderly or those in poor health, conversion to arthroplasty may be a better option after an initial attempt at ORIF of an intertrochanteric fracture. In a series, also reported by Haidukewych, 60 patients at a mean age of 78 years underwent revision to arthroplasty after failed treatment of an intertrochanteric hip fracture. The initial treatment of these fractures included 50 sliding hip screws, 3 cephalomedullary nails, 3 Jewett nails, 1 blade plate, 1 dynamic condylar screw, 1 fixation using 3 cannulated screws, and 1 that had been treated nonoperatively. Of these 60 patients, 32 underwent conversion to THA, 27 should received bipolar prosthesis, and 1 received a unipolar prosthesis. A variety of approaches were used including 33 anterolateral, 23 transtrochanteric, 4 posterior, and 3 staged procedures. The decision of total or hemiarthroplasty was made by the surgeon after evaluation of the acetabular cartilage. There were 5 reoperations including 1 revision of both components for aseptic loosening, 1 femoral component revision for aseptic loosening, 1 debridement, 1 rewiring of the greater trochanter, and 1 removal of a trochanteric cable. Overall survivorship in this series was 100% at 7 years and 89% at 10 years. Of the 44 patients who completed 2 years of follow-up, 39 had no or mild pain and 11 had moderate or severe pain, 40 of 44 were able to walk, and 26 used 1-arm support or less. Standard implants were used in 9 of 60 arthroplasty cases, 58% required calcar replacing stems, 5% needed increased neck prostheses, and 22% used long-stemmed prostheses without calcar replacement.

The outcomes of a series of failed sliding hip screws reported by Zhang[18] in 2004 also seem to be encouraging. Nineteen patients treated for intertrochanteric fracture with a sliding hip screw required revision to total or hemiarthroplasty; 15 of these patients completed 2 years of follow-up.

The average HHSs increased from 38.4 to 79.8. Nine had no pain, 3 reported mild pain, and 3 had slight occasional pain. Four patients could walk 6 or more blocks, 8 could walk 2 to 3 blocks, and 3 were limited to indoor ambulation. Two patients did not use an assistive device, 6 occasionally used a cane, 5 used a cane most of the time, and 3 used a walker.

In 2010, D'Arrigo[28] reported outcomes of 21 patients with failed intertrochanteric fracture fixation; 14 had failed nails, 5 had failed plates, 1 had a failed hip screw, and 1 had a failed Ender nail. In 19 patients the condition was salvaged with THA (18/19 press-fit) and 2 received bipolar implants. Fourteen were modular implants and 5 were standard THA implants. The minimum follow-up was 6 months. Preoperative Western Ontario and McMaster Universities Osteoarthritis Index (WOMAC) scores decreased from 87 to 47.3 at 1 month and to 40.8 at 6 months. The average HHS improved from 37 to 81. There were 4 of 21 patients with HHS between 90 and 100. Of the 21 patients, 10 scored from 80 to 89 and 2 scored from 70 to 79. There was 1 hip that rated poor and scored 65 on the Harris hip scoring system. Radiographically, there were no cases of loosening. One patient had died within 1 year with an intact implant.

Thakur[29] reported their results on using a cementless distally fitted stem for salvage of a failed intertrochanteric hip fracture; 15 patients underwent revision to THA (12) or bipolar implants (3). Their average follow-up was 2.86 years. At last follow-up, 3 patients used walkers, 10 used a cane, and 2 used no assistive devices. Two had residual trochanteric pain. However, the average HHS increased from 35.9 to 83.01. Of the total stems, 14 had bony ingrowth and 1 was undersized but stable. The mean limb length discrepancy was 2 mm (up to 5 mm short and 10 mm long).

The outcomes of salvage of failed trochanteric fractures using a curved cementless modular hip arthroplasty are also promising. In one series, 12 patients with failed sliding hip screw for intertrochanteric fracture and 4 for failed subtrochanteric fractures were salvaged to THA using this type of device. At mean follow-up of 60 months, 8 of 16 had complete pain relief and 8 of 16 reported minor trochanteric pain without compromise of activity. In this study, 8 used no assistive devices, 6 used a cane intermittently, and 2 used a cane most of the time. There was no loosening or subsidence. There was 1 patient with a greater trochanteric nonunion that migrated 15 mm and then stopped. The mean HHS improved from 17.8 to 87.7. They all had a Trendelenburg gait up to 6 months but recovered by 24 months.

SUMMARY

THA can be successfully performed in the setting of prior acetabular and proximal femoral fracture surgery with the expectation of excellent results. The complexity of the surgery and the rate of complications is increased compared with routine primary hip arthroplasty. Appropriate preoperative planning and awareness of the common complications can improve outcomes.

REFERENCES

1. Matta J. Fracture of the acetabulum: accuracy of reduction and clinical results in patients managed operatively within three weeks after the injury. J Bone Joint Surg Am 1996;78(11):1632–45.
2. Tannast M, Najibi S, Matta JM. Two to twenty-year survivorship of the hip in 810 patients with operatively treated acetabular fractures. J Bone Joint Surg Am 2012;94(17):1559–67.
3. Weber M, Berry DJ, Harmsen S. Total hip arthroplasty after operative treatment of acetabular fracture. J Bone Joint Surg Am 1998;80(9):1295–305.
4. Bellabarba C, Berger RA, Bentley CD, et al. Cementless acetabular reconstruction after acetabular fracture. J Bone Joint Surg Am 2001;83:868–76.
5. Berry DJ, Halasy M. Uncemented acetabular components for arthritis after acetabular fracture. Clin Orthop Relat Res 2002;(405):164–7.
6. Ranawat A, Zelken J, Helfet D, et al. Total hip arthroplasty for posttraumatic arthritis after acetabular fracture. J Arthroplasty 2009;24(5):759–66.
7. Sterling RS, Krushinski EM, Pellegrini VD. THA after acetabular fracture fixation: is frozen section necessary? Clin Orthop Relat Res 2011;469:547–51.
8. Zhang L, Zhou Y, Li Y. Total Hip Arthroplasty for failed treatment of acetabular fractures: a 5-year follow up survey. J Arthroplasty 2011;26(8):1189–93.
9. Haidukewych GJ, Rothwell WS, Jacofsky DJ, et al. Operative treatment of femoral neck fractures in patients between the ages of fifteen and fifty years. J Bone Joint Surg Am 2004;86-A(8):1711–6.
10. Asnis SE, Wanek-sgaglione L. Intracapsular fractures of the femoral neck. Results of cannulated screw fixation. J Bone Joint Surg Am 1994;76(12): 1793–803.
11. Franzen H, Nilsson LT, Stromqvist B, et al. Secondary total hip replacement after fractures of the femoral neck. J Bone Joint Surg Am 1990;72(5):784–7.
12. Santore RF, Turgeon TR, Phillips WF, et al. Pelvic and femoral osteotomy in the treatment of hip disease in the young adult. Instr Course Lect 2006;55:131–44.
13. Patterson BM, Salvati EA, Huo MH. Total hip arthroplasty for complications of intertrochanteric fracture: a technical note. J Bone Joint Surg Am 1990;72: 776–7.
14. Mehlhoff T, Landon GC, Tullos HS. Total hip arthroplasty following failed internal fixation of hip fractures. Clin Orthop Relat Res 1991;(269):32–7.
15. Stoffelen D, Haentjens P, Reynders P, et al. Hip arthroplasty for failed internal fixation of intertrochanteric and subtrochanteric fractures in the elderly patient. Acta Orthop Belg 1994;60:135–9.
16. Tabsh I, Waddell JP, Morton J. Total hip arthroplasty for complications of proximal femoral fractures. J Orthop Trauma 1997;11(3):166–9.
17. Haidukewych GJ, Berry D. Hip arthroplasty for salvage of failed treatment of intertrochanteric hip fractures. J Bone Joint Surg Am 2003;85:899–904.
18. Zhang B, Chiu K, Wang M. Hip arthroplasty for failed internal fixation of intertrochanteric fractures. J Arthroplasty 2004;19(3):329–33.
19. Kyle RF, Cooper J. Total hip arthroplasty after failed fixation of hip fractures. Orthopedics 2006;29(9):783–4.
20. Hernigou P, Poignard A, Mathieu G, et al. Total hip arthroplasty after failure of per- and subtrochanteric fracture fixation in elderly subjects. Rev Chir Orthop Reparatrice Appar Mot 2006;92(4):310–5.
21. Winemaker M, Gamble P, Petruccelli D, et al. Short-term outcomes of total hip arthroplasty after complications of open reduction internal fixation for hip fracture. J Arthroplasty 2006;21(5):682–8.
22. Said GZ, Farouk O, El-Sayed A, et al. Salvage of failed dynamic hip screw fixation of intertrochanteric fractures. Injury 2006;37:194–202.
23. Laffosse JM, Molinier F, Tricoire JL, et al. Cementless modular hip arthroplasty as a salvage operation for failed internal fixation of trochanteric fractures in elderly patients. Acta Orthop Belg 2007;73:729–36.
24. Lombardi AV, Skeels MD, Berend KR. Total hip arthroplasty after failed hip fracture: a challenging act. Orthopedics 2007;30(9):752–3.
25. Chen Y, Chen W, Lee K, et al. Diaphyseal locking hip arthroplasty for treatment of failed fixation of intertrochanteric hip fractures. J Arthroplasty 2008;23(2): 241–6.
26. Talmo CT, Bono JV. Treatment of intertrochanteric nonunion of the proximal femur using the S-ROM prosthesis. Orthopedics 2008;31(2):125.
27. Sharvill RJ, Ferran NA, Jones HG, et al. Long-stem revision prosthesis for salvage of failed fixation of extracapsular proximal femoral fractures. Acta Orthop Belg 2009;75:340–5.
28. D'Arrigo C, Perugia D, Carcangui A, et al. Hip arthroplasty for failed treatment of proximal femoral fractures. Int Orthop 2010;34:939–42.
29. Thakur RR, Deshmukh AJ, Goyal A, et al. Management of failed trochanteric fracture fixation with cementless modular hip arthroplasty using a distally fixing stem. J Arthroplasty 2011;26(3):398–403.
30. Abouelela AA. Salvage of failed trochanteric fracture fixation using the Revitan curved cementless modular hip arthroplasty. J Arthroplasty 2012;27(7):1382–8.

31. DeHaan AM, Tahnee G, Priddy M, et al. Salvage hip arthroplasty after failed fixation of proximal femur fractures. J Arthroplasty 2013;28:855–9.

32. Pui CM, Bostrom MP, Westrich GH, et al. Increased complication rate following conversion total hip arthroplasty after cephalomedullary fixation for intertrochanteric hip fracture: a multi-center study. J Arthroplasty 2013;28(8 Suppl):45–7.

33. Angelini M, McKee MD, Waddell JP, et al. Salvage of failed hip fracture fixation. J Orthop Trauma 2009; 23(6):471–8.

34. Mariani EM, Rand JA. Nonunion of intertrochanteric fractures of the femur following open reduction and internal fixation: results of second attempts to gain union. Clin Orthop Relat Res 1987;(218):81–9.

35. Wu CC, Shih CH, Chen WJ, et al. Treatment of cutout of a lag screw of a dynamic hip screw in an intertrochanteric fracture. Arch Orthop Trauma Surg 1998;117(4–5):193–6.

36. Haidukewych GJ, Berry D. Salvage of failed internal fixation of intertrochanteric hip fractures. Clin Orthop Relat Res 2003;(412):184–8.

37. Farrell CM, Springer BD, Haidukewych GJ, et al. Motor nerve palsy following primary total hip arthroplasty. J Bone Joint Surg Am 2005;87(12): 2619–25.

38. Bercik MJ, Miller AG, Muffly M, et al. Conversion total hip arthroplasty: a reason not to use cephalomedullary nails. J Arthroplasty 2012;27(8 Suppl): 117–21.

39. Mortazavi SM, Greenky MR, Bican O, et al. Total hip arthroplasty after prior surgical treatment of hip fracture: is it always challenging. J Arthroplasty 2012; 27(1):31–6.

A Growing Problem
Acetabular Fractures in the Elderly and the Combined Hip Procedure

Leonard T. Buller, MD[a,b], Charles M. Lawrie, MD[a,b], Fernando E. Vilella, MD[c,*]

KEYWORDS

- Acetabular fracture • Elderly • Combined hip procedure • Total hip arthroplasty

KEY POINTS

- The rate of acetabular fractures in the elderly is on the rise.
- Acetabular fractures in the elderly are more frequently caused by a low-energy mechanism, leading to characteristic fracture patterns.
- Geriatric patients often have multiple medical comorbidities and a multidisciplinary approach should be taken to their management.
- Acute total hip arthroplasty should be considered in a select group of elderly patients.

EPIDEMIOLOGY

As the elderly patient population continues to pursue more active lifestyles, the incidence of pelvic and acetabular fractures in the elderly is on the rise. Epidemiologic studies, starting in the 1970s, have demonstrated a steady increase in the global incidence of pelvic fractures sustained by individuals older than age 60.[1–3] This trend is expected to continue as the elderly population increases with 20% of the United States estimated to be older than the age of 65 years by 2030.[4] Kannus and colleagues[1] reviewed first time, low-energy, osteoporotic pelvic fractures in patients older than age 60 from the Finnish national trauma registry from 1970 through 1997. They found the number of elderly pelvic fractures increased by an average of 23% per year and the incidence of osteoporotic pelvic fractures as a percentage of all pelvic fractures increased from 18% to 64%.[1]

Similarly, Gansslen and colleagues[5] in a large, multicenter study from Germany reviewed 3260 patients of all ages with pelvic trauma and reported an increase in the incidence of pelvic trauma among patients aged 50 to 70 years from 1972 to 1993. The influence of age on the annual incidence of pelvic fractures cannot be overstated, because a four-fold increase is seen in patients greater than 80 years compared with 60 years of age.[6]

Fractures of the acetabulum in elderly individuals are the fastest growing segment of pelvic trauma.[7] Estimated to account for between 10% and 20% of all osteoporotic pelvic fractures,[8] the incidence of acetabular fractures has risen concurrent with all types of pelvic fractures in the geriatric age group.[9] Laird and Keating[2] demonstrated an increase in the average age of individuals with acetabular fractures from 1988 to 2003 at a single institution in Edinburgh, Scotland. In the United

The authors have nothing to disclose.

a Department of Orthopaedic Surgery, Jackson Memorial Hospital, University of Miami, 1400 Northwest 12th Avenue, Miami, FL 33136, USA; b Department of Rehabilitation, Jackson Memorial Hospital, University of Miami, 1400 Northwest 12th Avenue, Miami, FL 33136, USA; c Orthopaedic Trauma Service, Department of Orthopaedic Surgery, Ryder Trauma Center, Jackson Memorial Hospital, University of Miami, 1400 Northwest 12th Avenue, Miami, FL 33136, USA
* Corresponding author. Department of Orthopaedics, PO Box 016960 (D-27), Miami, FL 33101.
E-mail address: fvilella@med.miami.edu

States, Ferguson and colleagues[3] retrospectively reviewed records from 1980 to 2007 and found the percentage of displaced acetabular fractures in patients older than age 60 increased from 10% to 24% of the total number of displaced acetabular fractures in patients of all ages.

MECHANISM OF INJURY

Low-energy falls from standing height are the predominant mechanism of injury responsible for acetabular fractures in the elderly.[3,6] This is different from the typical high-energy trauma from motor vehicle accidents or from high falls that are responsible for most acetabular fractures seen in the younger population.[2,3] The positive correlation of age with fall from standing height resulting in injury is well known and thought to be the result of cognitive decline and motor impairment.[10] An estimated 30% of people older than age 65 and 40% of people older than age 80 fall and sustain an injury significant enough to warrant a visit to the emergency department annually.[11]

Importantly, when compared with younger individuals, seemingly low-energy falls cause significant injury and are the leading cause of injury-related death in the elderly population.[12] Sterling and colleagues[13] retrospectively reviewed data from a level two trauma center registry between 1994 and 1998 and found an injury severity score of greater than 15 in 30% of patients older than 65 compared with only 4% of patients younger than 65 who sustained a same level fall. The older cohort was more likely to sustain head, neck, chest, and pelvic injuries than the younger population and nearly twice as likely to die from a fall from any level.

ACETABULAR FRACTURE PATTERNS

Overall, associated both-column fractures are the most common acetabular fracture pattern observed in young and old individuals, accounting for 20% to 30% of acetabular fractures.[3,14] However, several unique features and fracture patterns are observed more commonly in elderly individuals, reflecting the difference in dominant mechanisms of injury.

Although high-energy trauma is responsible for most acetabular fractures in young patients, low-energy falls are the predominant mechanism of injury in the elderly, typically resulting in lateral compression type injuries.[8] The force from a direct impact on the greater trochanter is transmitted anteromedially to the anterior column, anterior wall, and quadrilateral plate. As a result, fractures of these structures are more common in the elderly

compared with younger individuals, who are more likely to sustain injury to the posterior column and wall and transverse patterns.[3,14,15] In the elderly, posterior wall involvement is more frequently associated with marginal impaction, comminution, and posterior hip dislocation than in young patients.[3,14] These features, and medial roof impaction, quadrilateral plate fracture, and injury to the femoral head, which are also seen at an increased rate in the elderly, are associated with poor outcomes after open reduction and internal fixation (ORIF) of acetabular fractures in the elderly.[3,14,16]

INITIAL EVALUATION

Even before arrival to the hospital, elderly patients are often undertriaged because of failure of emergency responders to recognize potential major injuries.[17] Several studies have demonstrated an increase in morbidity and mortality when elderly trauma patients are delayed in their arrival to a high-level trauma center.[9,18,19] Vital to every new clinical encounter, a thorough history should include assessment of the magnitude of the injury and the risk for concomitant injuries.[7] Specific to the elderly, assessment of comorbidities, preinjury ambulatory status, and life expectancy are essential during the initial assessment,[7,20] because they play a role in treatment decisions. The two most widely accepted and validated methods for assessment of comorbidities in the elderly population are the Charlson index[21] and the American Society of Anesthesiologists Classification (ASA) index.[20]

A high level of suspicion for severe injuries should be maintained during the evaluation of elderly patients, because they report less pain than younger patients for the same injury.[22] Additionally, when elderly patients do sustain high-energy trauma, they are significant more likely to be polytraumatized than younger patients.[12] Preexisting cognitive deficits, hearing difficulty, and other issues confound the use of the Glasgow Coma Scale in elderly patients.[23] Additionally, the initial trauma evaluation and physical examination of geriatric patients is different than for that of younger patients because of changes in their physiology, making evaluation and treatment difficult.[24] Specifically, vital signs considered within normal limits for younger patients, including heart rates greater than 90 beats per minute or systolic blood pressures less than 110 mm Hg, in the trauma setting, are associated with increased mortality in elderly patients.[25] Magnussen and colleagues[26] demonstrated that bleeding in acetabular fractures and age are directly correlated. Frequently lacking the cardiac reserve to adequately compensate, special attention should be paid to adequately resuscitating elderly patients to improve their chance of survival.[27]

Interdisciplinary approaches, with early involvement of geriatric specialists, have been shown to result in decreased hospital stays and reduced cost in protocol-driven programs for elderly patients with hip fractures.[28,29] In one study by Zuckerman and colleagues,[30] elderly patients with hip fractures treated in a multidisciplinary program were found to have fewer complications, fewer intensive care unit transfers, decreased mortality, improved ambulation, fewer discharges to long-term care facilities, and a 33% reduction in the cost of care when compared with age-matched control subjects not enrolled in the program.

DIAGNOSTIC IMAGING

Following initial assessment, patients with suspected pelvic trauma should undergo conventional radiographs consisting of anteroposterior, obturator, and iliac oblique views.[7] Frequently, patients undergo computed tomographic (CT) scan in their trauma work-up and the transaxial CT scan is useful in further fracture classification and for identifying acetabular impaction when section thickness is 3 mm or less.[7] Reformatted CT images in the sagittal or coronal plan are valuable for identifying central acetabular impaction,[7] whereas three-dimensional CT scans are useful for characterizing rotational deformities of the fragments.[31] Although most fractures can be identified easily with plain radiographs or CT scan, up to 5% of acetabular fractures are not detected on initial imaging.[32,33] When plain radiographs and CT scans fail to demonstrate pathology, but the clinical suspicion remains high, MRI and technetium bone scan have been found to have increased sensitivity in detecting nondisplaced insufficiency fractures common in osteoporotic bone.[34–36] In one study by Hakkarinen and colleagues[37] CT scan missed up to 20% of occult hip fractures that were subsequently detected on MRI, leading them to conclude that a negative CT scan is inadequate to exclude the diagnosis of acetabular fracture.

SURGICAL TIMING

The timing of surgery for acetabular fractures is a complex issue influenced by the resuscitation status of the patient, the fracture pattern and proposed surgical approach, and the requirement and availability of blood products.[15] Conflicting reports exist in the literature regarding exact timing of surgery for elderly patients and results of studies in younger patients. Vallier and colleagues[38]

demonstrated that early definitive fixation reduces morbidity and intensive care stay may not necessarily be generalizable to geriatric patients. Zuckerman and colleagues[39] found that delays of greater than 2 days resulted in a two-fold increase in mortality 1 year postoperatively. However, another study by Sexson and Lehner[40] evaluating patients with three or greater comorbidities found a lower survival rate in those treated within 24 hours of admission. Thus, preoperative evaluation and risk assessment by anesthesia and medicine are essential because elderly patients are susceptible to cardiac and pulmonary events, have decreased compensatory reserve, become coagulopathic more quickly, and have a higher risk of venous tears.[15] Because of the high risk of blood loss attributable to the size of the incision and difficulty in applying reduction clamps to osteoporotic bone,[15] the surgical team should be prepared for blood transfusion. Some purport the benefits of a cell saver machine,[15] although one study by Scannell and colleagues[41] demonstrated that there was no change in intraoperative and postoperative transfusion when cell saver was used during surgical management of acetabular fractures. The use of cell saver was, however, associated with higher total blood-related charges.[41]

TREATMENT

The treatment of acetabular fractures in the elderly is as varied as their presentation. Also, the heterogeneous nature of this specific population might complicate what is the optimal treatment of this injury. Other considerations include the capabilities of the treatment facility and the surgical skill of the treating surgeon. In the literature, there is a paucity of controlled, systemic reviews that might allow surgeons to reach adequate treatment conclusions. Options for the treatment of acetabular fractures in the elderly include nonoperative management; minimally invasive stabilization; conventional ORIF; delayed arthroplasty; or the combined hip procedure, which includes acute arthroplasty.

NONOPERATIVE MANAGEMENT

Nonoperative management should only be undertaken when it is expected to lead to good functional outcome with return to near preinjury activity level and not because no other options are available. This treatment strategy may be undertaken for several reasons pertaining to fracture pattern and patient factors:

- Minimally displaced, intrinsically stable injury patterns (eg, transverse type or anterior column fractures).

- Fractures with secondary congruence of the hip joint. This is frequently observed with both-column injuries where there is no continuity of the articular surface to the hemipelvis, but a congruent relationship is maintained between the femoral head and the acetabulum.[42]
- Significant medical comorbidities that contraindicate surgery.
- Severely limited preinjury mobility.

Several acetabular injury patterns have consistently demonstrated poor results with nonoperative management. In these cases, efforts should be made to perform surgical treatment whenever possible.

- Posterior instability caused by a large posterior wall fragment or posterior comminution. In these cases, even bed-to-chair transfers cause fracture displacement and possible hip dislocation because the moving from a recumbent to seated position forces the femoral head posteriorly against the unstable fracture.[43]
- Involvement of the weight-bearing dome.
- Quadrilateral plate impaction with medialization of the femoral head.

Nonoperative treatment should typically encompass bed-to-chair transfers followed by ambulation with assistance. Early mobilization is critical to avoid medical complications associated with prolonged recumbence. Strict bed rest is never indicated in management of these injuries. Partial weight-bearing should be initiated early on the affected extremity as tolerated. Although late displacement is uncommon if radiographs at 1 week are satisfactory, close radiographic follow-up should be performed to monitor for displacement, which may require a change in treatment strategy.[7]

Traction should not be used as definitive treatment of any acetabular fracture in the elderly. Hip capsular ligamentotaxis is unable to reliably correct the deforming forces that are typically rotational, not translational.[44] Additionally, a high rate of complications is observed, including medical issues from the requisite prolonged recumbence and pin site infections or pin pullout from osteoporotic bone.[45]

MINIMALLY INVASIVE FIXATION

Minimally invasive fixation of geriatric acetabular fractures is a technically challenging technique that may be used for a small subset of minimally displaced yet unstable fracture patterns. Using small stab incisions, modified clamps and ball spike pushers can be used to achieve reduction. Cannulated screws are then inserted in a percutaneous fashion.

Advantages of minimally invasive fixation include a reduced surgical physiologic insult versus traditional ORIF. This allows for surgical stabilization and early mobilization in a patient who otherwise might not be a candidate for a large open procedure.

It also makes future arthroplasty technically easier. Less scar tissue and soft tissue damage are present at the future surgical site, making the approach and dissection easier than if a formal ORIF had been performed. Additionally, reduction and stabilization of the fracture facilitate proper arthroplasty component positioning and fixation.

Disadvantages of minimally invasive fixation include limited access to the fracture site that leads to decreased ability to accurately anatomically reduce the fracture and apply stable hardware. Screw purchase in osteoporotic bone is unpredictable and it is technically challenging with safe zones for screw placement being small and complications from errant screw placement severe and life threatening.[46]

Despite the inability to achieve anatomic reduction with this technique in most cases, several series have reported that elderly patients may tolerate poor reductions better than their younger counterparts. Additionally, if malreduction leads to osteoarthritis, total hip arthroplasty remains a viable option in the elderly age group, which may not be an acceptable option in a younger patient. Most series to date have demonstrated equivalent outcomes with percutaneous fixation and open reduction with internal fixation; however, the authors note a large bias in patient selection for each type of procedure.[47–49]

CONVENTIONAL OPEN REDUCTION WITH INTERNAL FIXATION

ORIF remains standard care for most displaced acetabular fractures in the elderly. In most cases, it allows for direct fracture visualization and anatomic restoration of the joint surface that is a key factor for future prognosis. This is best achieved through a single, nonextensile approach in the elderly. Combined and extensile approaches should be avoided in this age group, because they have been associated with longer operative times and higher rates of complications.[50] However, occasionally they must be used to address displaced or comminuted articular fragments that cannot be otherwise addressed from a single, nonextensile approach.

For injuries involving posterior acetabulum or posterior column, a Kocher-Langenbeck approach is recommended. For those involving the anterior acetabulum or anterior column, an ilioinguinal approach is recommended.[51] For fractures involving both columns, an anterior or posterior approach is selected based on the acetabular column with the greatest displacement. The ilioinguinal approach has been the most widely used to address fractures of the quadrilateral plate.[16] However, a Stoppa approach or posterior-based approach may be considered based on certain fracture characteristics (**Fig. 1**).

After appropriate direct and indirect exposure of the fracture has been achieved, the specific techniques of reduction and fixation vary widely based on specific fracture pattern. However, several principles should be observed to give the best chance of an optimal outcome. First, in the osteoporotic bone typically seen in elderly patients, lag screws alone should not be relied on for stable fixation and should be supplemented with at least one buttress plate for wall fractures and neutralization plates for column fractures.[52] In fractures of the quadrilateral plate, careful attention must be paid to proper reduction and neutralization of the medial fragment protrusion, and/or any impaction that may be present.[16] Optimal overall outcome may be achieved with nonanatomic reduction while still providing adequate reduction and fixation of the columns to allow for healing and early mobilization, because the degree of comminution and poor bone stock often encountered in the elderly patient can make true anatomic reduction difficult if not impossible to achieve without increasing morbidity with prolonged operative times and large exposures.[7]

Several predictors of clinical outcome after ORIF of displaced elderly acetabular fractures have been consistently demonstrated. Factors that predict poor outcome include posterior wall fracture with an associated posterior hip dislocation, comminution or marginal impaction,[53] femoral head injury,[54,55] and quadrilateral plate involvement.[16]

Outcomes of ORIF of elderly acetabular fractures are notoriously worse than those in the younger population. A large systematic review of acetabular fractures in patients aged greater than 55 years found ORIF resulted in anatomic reduction in 45.3% and conversion to total hip arthroplasty of 23.1% compared with approximately

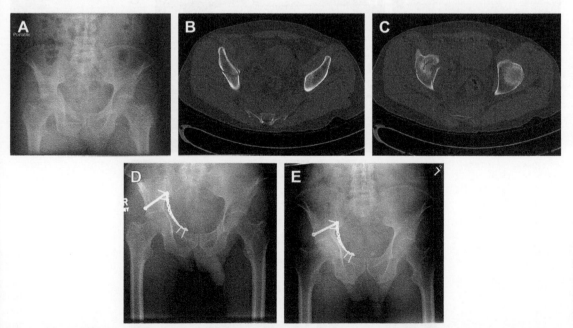

Fig. 1. Case of a 65-year-old man who fell of his bicycle at a low rate of speed with trauma to the right hip. (*A*) Plain radiographs demonstrate quadrilateral surface involvement and protrusion. Computerized tomography with evidence of (*B*) fracture through the anterior column, and (*C*) a more distal cut demonstrating a low both-column pattern with involvement of the quadrilateral surface. (*D*) The fracture was treated with traditional open reduction and internal fixation through a modified Stoppa approach, with percutaneous screw placement for the anterior column and infrapectineal buttress plating of the quadrilateral surface. (*E*) Radiographs at 2 years postsurgery demonstrate adequate healing and no arthrosis. Patient had no pain and returned to full activity level.

75% anatomic reduction rate and conversion to total hip arthroplasty around 8% in younger patients.[14]

NONOPERATIVE MANAGEMENT WITH DELAYED TOTAL HIP ARTHROPLASTY

Select elderly patients with acetabular fractures may develop posttraumatic arthritis or avascular necrosis of the femoral head, leading to a painful hip joint.[50] Regardless of the initial management method[43,56] total hip arthroplasty may be necessary. Factors placing patients at a higher risk of requiring an arthroplasty include radiographic features that predict poor outcome, initial mechanism of injury, type of fracture, age and weight of patient, time from injury, and initial management strategy.[50,56,57]

The basic tenet of nonoperative management with delayed total hip arthroplasty after an acetabular fracture involves the concept of performing a hip arthroplasty in soft tissue that has not received a previous surgical insult (**Fig. 2**). However, in patients treated nonoperatively,

residual displacement leading to misalignment of the acetabulum, the presence of osseous defects, or nonunion of the acetabulum may impede a consequent arthroplasty and necessitate use of bone grafts or cages.[58]

Multiple surgical approaches exist to correct the variety of anatomic and pathologic problems among elderly patients with posttraumatic arthritis.[59–64] Most standard surgical approaches include a posterior approach or an anterolateral Hardinge approach.[64] With significant deformity or heterotopic bone, modified approaches may be necessary. Options include Kocher-Langenbeck approach[56] for patients with a fractured posterior wall or column, triradiate incision with preservation of the greater trochanter for visualization of the anterior and posterior aspect of the acetabulum and hip joint,[65] and extended iliofemoral approach when there is involvement of the entire hemipelvis and corrective osteotomies are part of the arthroplasty.[50]

In patients with combined acetabular and pelvic ring injuries, correction of the pelvic ring alignment is necessary before the arthroplasty, with a variety

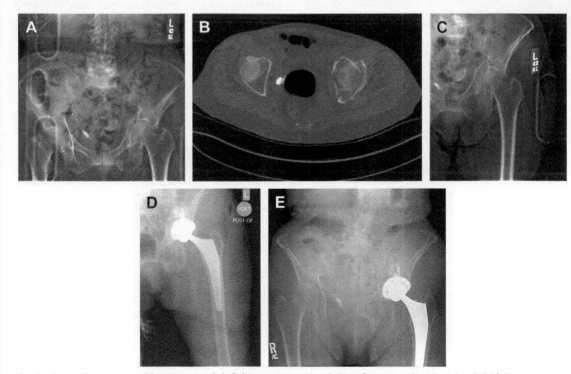

Fig. 2. Case of a 79-year-old woman with left hip trauma after falling from standing height. (*A*) Plain anteroposterior pelvis radiographs demonstrate a left acetabular fracture with significant comminution and protrusion. (*B*) CT shows comminution and a low both-column fracture pattern. The patient was acutely treated with nonoperative management. (*C*) One-year radiograph with evidence of fracture healing, essentially in the same position. (*D*) The patient was ambulating with significant pain and a delayed arthroplasty was performed with lateralization of the hip center. (*E*) One year later, the implant was well fixed and the patient was ambulating with minimal difficulty.

of described techniques.[50] In patients with significant bone defects, a ring or cage with various extension plates[59,60] is in use. Cages act as a form of internal fixation that immobilizes sites of nonunion, with supplementary bone graft filling in any gaps that remain between the surface of the cage and the pelvis.[50] Despite the benefits of cages in patients who lack bone stock, risks include the potential for loosening of the screws or the cage when anchored in osteopenic bone. Recently, metal-backed polyethylene liners that secure to the cage have decreased the use of bone cement.[50] On the femoral side, cemented and cementless stems are available.[66] Studies evaluating total hip arthroplasty performed following an acetabular fracture have documented a high rate of premature loosening among patients receiving cementless stems.[67–70] The authors hypothesize that the period of inactivity and restricted weight-bearing following the injury and after the development of osteoarthritis leads to a disuse osteoporosis[50] and predisposes patients to premature loosening. Consequently, they suggest that these patients should undergo cemented stems.[50]

OPEN REDUCTION AND INTERNAL FIXATION WITH DELAYED ARTHROPLASTY

As with any acetabular fracture requiring ORIF, the goal of operative management is to restore the anatomy of the acetabulum so as to delay the onset of posttraumatic arthritis. ORIF can be acute or delayed,[71] with the delayed strategy valuable for younger patients with simple fracture patterns and no evidence of significant impaction.[50] Patients presenting with posttraumatic arthritis following surgical fixation of an acetabular fracture are often candidates for total hip arthroplasty. Delayed arthroplasty following ORIF is made more difficult because of the presence of scar tissue, disruptive hardware, heterotopic bone, avascularity of soft tissue and bone, and a possible occult infection.[67]

Outcomes following delayed arthroplasty for posttraumatic arthritis are less favorable than for patients undergoing arthroplasty for primary degenerative joint disease,[68,70,72,73] with revision rates up to 20-fold higher.[50] In one study, the rate of radiographic loosening was 53% and 14% required revision.[68] In another study by Stauffer,[73] 37% had radiographic evidence of loosening and the revision rate was 8%.

COMBINED HIP PROCEDURE

Because of the poor outcomes reported with delayed arthroplasty for posttraumatic arthritis

following acetabular fracture, investigators have begun developing strategies for acutely performing total hip arthroplasty.[50] The combined hip procedure involves operative stabilization of an acetabular fracture with acute placement of a total hip arthroplasty. The rationale of this procedure is that a single surgery can be performed for those geriatric acetabular fractures that have an unfavorable prognosis and have the strong chance of needing conversion to arthroplasty at a later date. Indications for the combined hip procedure include presence of a femoral neck fracture or significant damage to the femoral head including femoral head abrasions, impaction, or fracture; severe, unreconstructible acetabular comminution and impaction involving 30% of its surface; pre-existing hip arthrosis; multiple associated fractures; and those who have a low likelihood for a satisfactory outcome following ORIF, and in whom ORIF has been shown to compromise the success of a subsequent arthroplasty (**Fig. 3**).[50] Ideal patient factors for the combined hip procedure are osteopenic bone, advanced age, patients with substantial medical comorbidities, and when there is a significant delay from injury to surgery.[50] In very elderly patients with significantly osteopenic bone and substantial fracture displacement, the risks and benefits to acute arthroplasty should be carefully weighed.

The combined hip procedure can typically be performed through a single Kocher-Lagenbeck approach, but anterior fixation should be done through an anterior approach if necessary. After the femoral neck cut, the entire acetabulum can be visualized, which allows the surgeon to optimally stabilize the fracture, with the appropriate combination of plates and screws that creates a stable construct. The purpose of reducing and stabilizing the acetabular fracture is not necessarily to achieve an anatomic reduction, but rather to create a stable construct for placement of the cup. Acetabular reaming should be undertaken in a very controlled, gentle fashion because of the soft quality of the bone, with little medicalization. Any deficiency of the posterior wall or any portion of the wall that is unreconstructible can be addressed by using the femoral head as autograft. This is performed by cutting away the inferior portion of the head into a "seven" pattern, then fixing it to the posterior column with interfragmentary lag screws and/or buttressing plating. A multi-hole cup should be used routinely so it serves as additional fixation within the reconstructed acetabulum. The femoral component is done in standard fashion with either press fit or cemented techniques depending on patient age, bone quality, or surgeon preference. The patient should

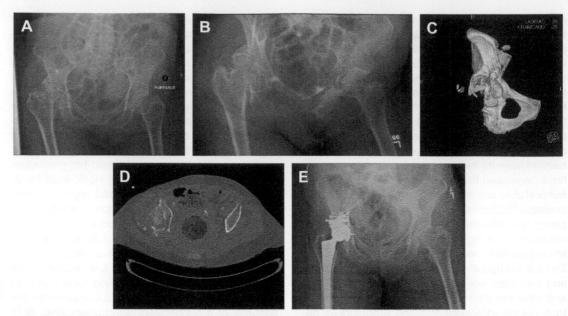

Fig. 3. Case of a 72-year-old woman involved in a motor vehicle collision 1 week before admission at our trauma center. (*A*) Anteroposterior pelvic radiograph demonstrating a right acetabular fracture with subluxation of the femoral head. (*B*) Obturator oblique radiograph with a comminuted posterior wall fracture. (*C*) Three-dimensional CT of the fracture with severe comminution of the posterior wall. (*D*) The combination of fracture comminution and her osteopenic bone made posterior wall unreconstructible. The patient's native femoral head was used as autograft reconstruction and stabilized to the pelvis, and a total hip arthroplasty (*E*) was performed.

be placed into an abduction bolster postoperatively.[50] In most cases, bed-to-chair transfers can be initiated on postoperative Day 1. Light partial weight-bearing can begin on postoperative Day 2 with progression to full weight-bearing at 6 to 8 weeks.[50]

Outcomes following acute arthroplasty for an acetabular fracture have been generally good with low complication rates.[7,50,65] In a series by Mears and Velyvis,[65] 57 patients with an average follow-up of 8.1 years demonstrated an 89% healing rate at 12 weeks, with 79% of patients having excellent or good Harris Hip Scores. They did report, however, between 2 and 3 mm of acetabular component displacement. There were no cases of deep infection and no cases of radiographic or symptomatic femoral loosening. Their conclusion was that the combined hip procedure seemed to be a successful procedure in the elderly. Herscovici and colleagues[74] published a series of 22 patients with an average age of 75.3 years with an average follow-up of 29.4 months. All surgeries were performed in a single setting, and in general their data with regard to the combined hip procedure was comparable with that from acetabular revision surgery. Four of their patients (18%) had revisions, two for acetabular loosening, and two for irreducible dislocation.

The series by Boraiah and colleagues[75] included 21 patients with an average age of 72 and 3.9 years of follow-up. Eighty-one percent of these patients had excellent or good Harris Hip Scores, with one revision (5%) caused by recurrent dislocation. Chakravarty and colleagues[76] published a series of 19 patients, with an average age of 77 years, where stabilization of the acetabular fracture was achieved through minimally invasive techniques, with acute placement of a total hip arthroplasty. This technique avoided extensive surgical approaches, minimized soft tissue complications, and at the same time provided column stability with early pain relief and mobilization through immediate arthroplasty.

Variations in technique include that published by Rickman and colleagues[77] where the anterior column and the posterior column were plated through different approaches, creating an A-frame with the cup as the crosspiece. A trabecular metal cup was placed in whatever position achieved maximal stability, and then the liner was cemented in proper orientation. The initial stability of the trabecular metal cup, its properties of osseous integration, and the mechanical stability of the A-frame allowed early mobilization and weight-bearing as tolerated, which is critical in the elderly population. Other technical variations include the acute use of cages. Malhotra and colleagues[78] had a series of 15 patients, with an average age of 64.5 years, all treated with a posterior approach with ORIF of the fracture then placement of bone graft, a cementless cup, and liner. All patients were weight-bearing as tolerated by 6 weeks, with 87% excellent or good Harris Hip Scores, and no evidence of cup migration or osteolysis. They concluded that their cage allows correct placement of the center of rotation, initial stability that allows early weight-bearing, and the large contact area with bone graft allows good osseous integration, and no migration. Chana-Rodriguez and coworkers[79] used a cup-cage construct in their series of six patients. They used a single, posterior approach with placement of a cage, graft, a trabecular metal cup, and then the liner was cemented into the desired position. Only one component medialized and 83% of patients had excellent-to-good results with Merle d'Aubinge-Postel Scoring. This was presented as a novel indication for a cup-cage construct, applying revision surgery techniques to achieve an acute, stable reconstruction that allows early weight-bearing.

SUMMARY

Acetabular fractures in the elderly are on the rise, and the variations in their management represent a growing problem within the orthopedic community. Fracture patterns are different in this population, with particular regard to low, anterior column involvement and significant, posterior comminution that poses a limitation on reconstruction. The combined hip procedure is a therapeutic option in this patient population, and its indications and techniques continue to evolve.

REFERENCES

1. Kannus P, Palvanen M, Niemi S, et al. Epidemiology of osteoporotic pelvic fractures in elderly people in Finland: sharp increase in 1970-1997 and alarming projections for the new millennium. Osteoporos Int 2000;11(5):443–8.

2. Laird A, Keating JF. Acetabular fractures: a 16-year prospective epidemiological study. J Bone Joint Surg Br 2005;87(7):969–73.

3. Ferguson TA, Patel R, Bhandari M, et al. Fractures of the acetabulum in patients aged 60 years and older: an epidemiological and radiological study. J Bone Joint Surg Br 2010;92(2):250–7.

4. Centers for Disease Control and Prevention. The state of aging & health in America 2013. In: Centers for Disease Control and Prevention. US Dept of Health and Human Services; 2013.

5. Gansslen A, Pohlemann T, Paul C, et al. Epidemiology of pelvic ring injuries. Injury 1996;27(Suppl 1):S-A13–20.

6. Krappinger D, Kammerlander C, Hak DJ, et al. Low-energy osteoporotic pelvic fractures. Arch Orthop Trauma Surg 2010;130(9):1167–75.

7. Mears DC. Surgical treatment of acetabular fractures in elderly patients with osteoporotic bone. J Am Acad Orthop Surg 1999;7(2):128–41.

8. Callaway DW, Wolfe R. Geriatric trauma. Emerg Med Clin North Am 2007;25(3):837–60, x.

9. Meldon SW, Reilly M, Drew BL, et al. Trauma in the very elderly: a community-based study of outcomes at trauma and nontrauma centers. J Trauma 2002; 52(1):79–84.

10. Campbell AJ, Robertson MC, Gardner MM, et al. Randomised controlled trial of a general practice programme of home based exercise to prevent falls in elderly women. BMJ 1997;315(7115):1065–9.

11. Prudham D, Evans JG. Factors associated with falls in the elderly: a community study. Age Ageing 1981; 10(3):141–6.

12. Switzer JA, Gammon SR. High-energy skeletal trauma in the elderly. J Bone Joint Surg Am 2012; 94(23):2195–204.

13. Sterling DA, O'Connor JA, Bonadies J. Geriatric falls: injury severity is high and disproportionate to mechanism. J Trauma 2001;50(1):116–9.

14. Daurka JS, Pastides PS, Lewis A, et al. Acetabular fractures in patients aged > 55 years: a systematic review of the literature. Bone Joint J 2014;96-B(2): 157–63.

15. Hill BW, Switzer JA, Cole PA. Management of high-energy acetabular fractures in the elderly individuals: a current review. Geriatr Orthop Surg Rehabil 2012;3(3):95–106.

16. White G, Kanakaris NK, Faour O, et al. Quadrilateral plate fractures of the acetabulum: an update. Injury 2013;44(2):159–67.

17. Phillips S, Rond PC III, Kelly SM, et al. The failure of triage criteria to identify geriatric patients with trauma: results from the Florida Trauma Triage Study. J Trauma 1996;40(2):278–83.

18. Lehmann R, Beekley A, Casey L, et al. The impact of advanced age on trauma triage decisions and outcomes: a statewide analysis. Am J Surg 2009; 197(5):571–4 [discussion: 574–5].

19. Shifflette VK, Lorenzo M, Mangram AJ, et al. Should age be a factor to change from a level II to a level I trauma activation? J Trauma 2010;69(1):88–92.

20. Guerado E, Cano JR, Cruz E. Fractures of the acetabulum in elderly patients: an update. Injury 2012; 43(Suppl 2):S33–41.

21. Charlson ME, Pompei P, Ales KL, et al. A new method of classifying prognostic comorbidity in longitudinal studies: development and validation. J Chronic Dis 1987;40(5):373–83.

22. Gibson SJ, Helme RD. Age-related differences in pain perception and report. Clin Geriatr Med 2001; 17(3):433–56, v–vi.

23. Zuercher M, Ummenhofer W, Baltussen A, et al. The use of Glasgow Coma Scale in injury assessment: a critical review. Brain Inj 2009;23(5):371–84.

24. Bonne S, Schuerer DJ. Trauma in the older adult: epidemiology and evolving geriatric trauma principles. Clin Geriatr Med 2013;29(1):137–50.

25. Heffernan DS, Thakkar RK, Monaghan SF, et al. Normal presenting vital signs are unreliable in geriatric blunt trauma victims. J Trauma 2010;69(4): 813–20.

26. Magnussen RA, Tressler MA, Obremskey WT, et al. Predicting blood loss in isolated pelvic and acetabular high-energy trauma. J Orthop Trauma 2007; 21(9):603–7.

27. Scalea TM, Simon HM, Duncan AO, et al. Geriatric blunt multiple trauma: improved survival with early invasive monitoring. J Trauma 1990;30(2):129–34 [discussion: 134–6].

28. Kates SL, Mendelson DA, Friedman SM. The value of an organized fracture program for the elderly: early results. J Orthop Trauma 2011;25(4):233–7.

29. Ceder L, Thorngren KG, Wallden B. Prognostic indicators and early home rehabilitation in elderly patients with hip fractures. Clin Orthop Relat Res 1980;(152):173–84.

30. Zuckerman JD, Sakales SR, Fabian DR, et al. Hip fractures in geriatric patients. Results of an interdisciplinary hospital care program. Clin Orthop Relat Res 1992;(274):213–25.

31. Haidukewych GJ. Acetabular fractures: the role of arthroplasty. Orthopedics 2010;33(9). http://dx.doi.org/10.3928/01477447-20100722-33.

32. Evans PD, Wilson C, Lyons K. Comparison of MRI with bone scanning for suspected hip fracture in elderly patients. J Bone Joint Surg Br 1994;76(1): 158–9.

33. Dominguez S, Liu P, Roberts C, et al. Prevalence of traumatic hip and pelvic fractures in patients with suspected hip fracture and negative initial standard radiographs: a study of emergency department patients. Acad Emerg Med 2005;12(4):366–9.

34. Tornkvist H, Schatzker J. Acetabular fractures in the elderly: an easily missed diagnosis. J Orthop Trauma 1993;7(3):233–5.

35. Lubovsky O, Liebergall M, Mattan Y, et al. Early diagnosis of occult hip fractures MRI versus CT scan. Injury 2005;36(6):788–92.

36. Koval KJ, Zuckerman JD. Functional recovery after fracture of the hip. J Bone Joint Surg Am 1994; 76(5):751–8.

37. Hakkarinen DK, Banh KV, Hendey GW. Magnetic resonance imaging identifies occult hip fractures missed by 64-slice computed tomography. J Emerg Med 2012;43(2):303–7.

38. Vallier HA, Cureton BA, Ekstein C, et al. Early definitive stabilization of unstable pelvis and acetabulum fractures reduces morbidity. J Trauma 2010;69(3): 677–84.

39. Zuckerman JD, Skovron ML, Koval KJ, et al. Postoperative complications and mortality associated with operative delay in older patients who have a fracture of the hip. J Bone Joint Surg Am 1995; 77(10):1551–6.

40. Sexson SB, Lehner JT. Factors affecting hip fracture mortality. J Orthop Trauma 1987;1(4):298–305.

41. Scannell BP, Loeffler BJ, Bosse MJ, et al. Efficacy of intraoperative red blood cell salvage and autotransfusion in the treatment of acetabular fractures. J Orthop Trauma 2009;23(5):340–5.

42. Gansslen A, Hildebrand F, Krettek C. Conservative treatment of acetabular both column fractures: does the concept of secondary congruence work? Acta Chir Orthop Traumatol Cech 2012;79(5):411–5.

43. Tile M. Fractures of the pelvis and acetabulum. Baltimore (MD): Williams and Wilkins; 1995. p. 176–84.

44. Matta JM, Mehne DK, Roffi R. Fractures of the acetabulum. Early results of a prospective study. Clin Orthop Relat Res 1986;(205):241–50.

45. Spencer RF. Acetabular fractures in older patients. J Bone Joint Surg Br 1989;71(5):774–6.

46. Puchwein P, Enninghorst N, Sisak K, et al. Percutaneous fixation of acetabular fractures: computer-assisted determination of safe zones, angles and lengths for screw insertion. Arch Orthop Trauma Surg 2012;132(6):805–11.

47. Gary JL, Lefaivre KA, Gerold F, et al. Survivorship of the native hip joint after percutaneous repair of acetabular fractures in the elderly. Injury 2011; 42(10):1144–51.

48. Gary JL, VanHal M, Gibbons SD, et al. Functional outcomes in elderly patients with acetabular fractures treated with minimally invasive reduction and percutaneous fixation. J Orthop Trauma 2012; 26(5):278–83.

49. Starr AJ, Jones AL, Reinert CM, et al. Preliminary results and complications following limited open reduction and percutaneous screw fixation of displaced fractures of the acetabulum. Injury 2001; 32(Suppl 1):SA45–50.

50. Mears DC, Velyvis JH. Primary total hip arthroplasty after acetabular fracture; an instructional course lecture, American Academy of Orthopaedic Surgeons. Bone Joint J 2000;82(9):1328.

51. Jeffcoat DM, Carroll EA, Huber FG, et al. Operative treatment of acetabular fractures in an older population through a limited ilioinguinal approach. J Orthop Trauma 2012;26(5):284–9.

52. Helfet DL, Borrelli J Jr, DiPasquale T, et al. Stabilization of acetabular fractures in elderly patients. J Bone Joint Surg Am 1992;74(5):753–65.

53. Kreder HJ, Rozen N, Borkhoff CM, et al. Determinants of functional outcome after simple and complex acetabular fractures involving the posterior wall. J Bone Joint Surg Br 2006;88(6):776–82.

54. Zha GC, Sun JY, Dong SJ. Predictors of clinical outcomes after surgical treatment of displaced acetabular fractures in the elderly. J Orthop Res 2013; 31(4):588–95.

55. Anglen JO, Burd TA, Hendricks KJ, et al. The "Gull Sign": a harbinger of failure for internal fixation of geriatric acetabular fractures. J Orthop Trauma 2003;17(9):625–34.

56. Letournel E, Judet R. Fractures of the acetabulum. 2nd edition. New York: Springer; 1993. p. 359–86.

57. Matta JM. Fractures of the acetabulum: accuracy of reduction and clinical results in patients managed operatively within three weeks after the injury. J Bone Joint Surg Am 1996;78(11):1632–45.

58. Mears DC, Rubash HE. Pelvic and acetabular fractures. Thorofare (NJ): Slack; 1986. p. 422–39.

59. Peters CL, Curtain M, Samuelson KM. Acetabular revision with the Burch-Schnieder antiprotrusio cage and cancellous allograft bone. J Arthroplasty 1995;10(3):307–12.

60. Moed BR. Acetabular fractures: the Kocher-Langenbeck approach. In: Wiss DA, editor. Master techniques in orthopaedic surgery. Philadelphia: Lippincott-Raven; 1998. p. 631–55.

61. Matta JM, Reilly MC. Acetabular fractures: the ilioinguinal approach. In: Wiss DA, editor. Master techniques in orthopaedic surgery. Philadelphia: Lippincott-Raven; 1998. p. 657–73.

62. Helfet DL, Bartlett CS, Malkani AL. Acetabular fractures: the extended iliofemoral approach. In: Wiss DA, editor. Fractures: master techniques in orthopaedic surgery. Philadelphia: Lippincott-Raven; 1998. p. 675–95.

63. Mears DC, MacLeod MD. Acetabular fractures: the triradiate and modified triradiate approaches. In: Wiss DA, editor. Fractures: master techniques in orthopaedic surgery. Philadelphia: Lippincott-Raven; 1998. p. 697–724.

64. Hardinge K. The direct lateral approach to the hip. J Bone Joint Surg Br 1982;64(1):17–9.

65. Mears DC, Velyvis JH. Acute total hip arthroplasty for selected displaced acetabular fractures: two to twelve-year results. J Bone Joint Surg Am 2002;84-A(1):1–9.

66. Galante JO. Overview of total hip arthroplasty. In: Callaghan J, Rosenberg A, Rubash H, editors. The adult hip. Philadelphia: Lippincott-Raven; 1998. p. 829–38.

67. Jimenez ML, Tile M, Schenk RS. Total hip replacement after acetabular fracture. Orthop Clin North Am 1997;28(3):435–46.

68. Romness DW, Lewallen DG. Total hip arthroplasty after fracture of the acetabulum. Long-term results. J Bone Joint Surg Br 1990;72(5):761–4.

69. Sim FH, Stauffer RN. Management of hip fractures by total hip arthroplasty. Clin Orthop Relat Res 1980;(152):191–7.

70. Weber M, Berry DJ, Harmsen WS. Total hip arthroplasty after operative treatment of an acetabular fracture. J Bone Joint Surg Am 1998;80(9):1295–305.

71. Johnson EE, Matta JM, Mast JW, et al. Delayed reconstruction of acetabular fractures 21-120 days following injury. Clin Orthop Relat Res 1994;(305): 20–30.

72. Carnesale PG, Stewart MJ, Barnes SN. Acetabular disruption and central fracture-dislocation of the hip. A long-term study. J Bone Joint Surg Am 1975;57(8):1054–9.

73. Stauffer RN. Ten-year follow-up study of total hip replacement. J Bone Joint Surg Am 1982;64(7): 983–90.

74. Herscovici D, Lindvall E, Bolhofner B, et al. The combined hip procedure: open reduction and internal fixation combined with total hip arthroplasty for the management of acetabular fractures in the elderly. J Orthop Trauma 2010;24(5):291–6.

75. Boraiah S, Ragsdale M, Achor T, et al. Open reduction and internal fixation and primary total hip arthroplasty of selected acetabular fractures. J Orthop Trauma 2009;23(4):243–8.

76. Chakravarty R, Toosi N, Katsman A, et al. Percutaneous column fixation and total hip arthroplasty for the treatment of acute acetabular fracture in the elderly. J Arthroplasty 2014;29:817–21.

77. Rickman M, Young J, Trompeter A, et al. Managing Acetabular fractures in the elderly with fixation and primary arthroplasty. Clin Orthop Relat Res 2014; 472(11):3375–82.

78. Malhotra R, Singh DP, Jain V, et al. Acute total hip arthroplasty in acetabular fractures in the elderly using the octopus system mid term to long term follow up. J Arthroplasty 2013;28:1005–9.

79. Chana-Rodriguez F, Villanueva-Martinez M, Rojo-Manaute J, et al. Cup cage construct for acute fractures of the acetabulum, redefining indications. Injury 2012;43(S2):S28–32.

Uses of Negative Pressure Wound Therapy in Orthopedic Trauma

Mark J. Gage, MD[a], Richard S. Yoon, MD[a],
Kenneth A. Egol, MD[a], Frank A. Liporace, MD[a,b],*

KEYWORDS

- Negative pressure wound therapy • VAC • Infection • Trauma • Open wound • Wound dehiscence
- Limb salvage • Open fracture

KEY POINTS

- Negative pressure wound therapy (NPWT) is ideal for soft tissue defects that can heal through secondary intention or require skin grafting.
- NPWT prevents desiccation, reduces edema, limits hematoma, and facilitates wound drainage.
- NPWT is an effective way to downscale the complexity of soft tissue reconstruction.
- NPWT can decreases the risk of wound complication when applied to high-risk incisions after fracture surgery.

INTRODUCTION

Since its inception more than 20 years ago, negative pressure wound therapy (NPWT) has had a major impact in the management of orthopedic injuries. NPWT has been widely adopted for use in a variety of clinical scenarios, and has had reported success in the setting of high-energy trauma, open fractures, infections, and excessive soft tissue damage. However, although its success has led to widespread use in orthopedic trauma, a deeper understanding of its mechanism of action, along with the ideal clinical scenarios for use, is required. This article reviews the nuances of NPWT application, including its mechanism of action, clinical indications, and specific strategies used in order to achieve desired clinical outcomes.

WHAT IS IT?

To administer NPWT, there are 3 main components that create a subatmospheric pressure environment: a porous dressing sealed via an occlusive adhesive, a vacuum device, and a connector that allows communication (**Fig. 1**). In orthopedic trauma, the dressing of choice is a dry, black, hydrophobic, reticulated polyurethane-ether foam with a pore size of 400 to 600 μm (KCI, San Antonio, TX). A polyvinyl alcohol (PVA) foam is also available (KCI, San Antonio, TX). It differs from the large-pore foam because it has a smaller pore size (60–270 μm) and comes premoistened with sterile water. The hydrophilic nature and smaller pore size of the PVA foam offers a less-adherent application and has significantly less granulation and perfusion than the large-pore dressing.[1] Thus, for

Conflicts of interest: The authors report no conflict of interest.
[a] Division of Orthopaedic Trauma, Department of Orthopaedic Surgery, NYU Hospital for Joint Diseases, New York, NY, USA; [b] Orthopaedic Trauma and Adult Reconstruction, Department of Orthopaedic Surgery, Jersey City Medical Center, 377 Jersey Avenue, Suite 220, Jersey City, NJ 07302, USA
* Corresponding author. Orthopaedic Trauma Research, Division of Orthopaedic Trauma, Department of Orthopaedic Surgery, NYU Hospital for Joint Diseases, New York, NY.
E-mail address: liporace33@gmail.com

Orthop Clin N Am 46 (2015) 227–234
http://dx.doi.org/10.1016/j.ocl.2014.11.002
0030-5898/15/$ – see front matter © 2015 Elsevier Inc. All rights reserved.

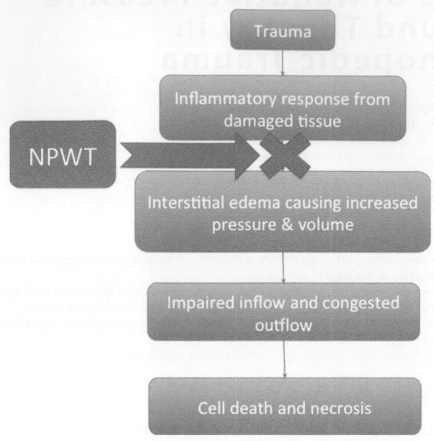

Fig. 1. NPWT disrupts the inflammatory cascade by reducing edema, limiting hematoma, and facilitating wound drainage to augment wound healing.

most of the clinical scenarios in orthopedic trauma, the large-pore foam is preferred. Placed on the area of interest, the wound and sponge dressing are sealed off with a plastic adhesive and occlusive dressing, and communicate with the vacuum device via a connector creating a localized negative pressure environment.

HOW DOES IT WORK?

NPWT allows improved wound management and healing via 2 main mechanisms. Following initial injury, a substantial inflammatory response is generated from damaged tissue, initiating a vicious cycle of increasing interstitial edema and pressure, leading to cell death and necrosis secondary to lack of nutrient inflow combined with a congested outflow of cellular waste (see **Fig. 1**). With the use of NPWT, a subatmospheric environment is created, acting at the level of the interstitium to eliminate unwanted edema, inflammatory mediators, and bacteria (see **Fig. 1**). This environment creates more favorable healing conditions by removing the volume that obstructs inflow and

outflow, allowing greater nutrient and oxygen inflow as well as venous drainage.[2]

In addition, NPWT promotes mitogenesis and granulation tissue formation via increased cellular substrate recruitment. Dynamic tissue formation is facilitated by the mechanical strain placed on the tissue by the negative pressure environment. The strain created by the vacuum allows microdeformation and stretch at the cellular level, allowing cellular chemotaxis, angiogenesis, and new tissue formation via the recruitment of growth factors (ie, vascular endothelial growth factor [VEGF], Fibroblastic Growth Factor [FGF]-2).[3,4] Labler and colleagues[3] analyzed wound fluid from NPWT dressings and noted significantly higher levels of interleukin-8 and VEGF compared with fluid analyzed from a standard dressing. Furthermore, histologic analysis noted significantly higher levels of angiogenesis and granulation tissue formation.

The effect of the subatmospheric environment is also evident at the genetic transcriptional level. Chen and colleagues[5] measured the presence of proto-oncogenes during NPWT in a pig model. The negative pressure environments produced significantly higher levels of C-MYC, C-JUN, and BCL-2, corresponding with proportional increases in the cells required for granulation tissue formation.[4] These cellular-level changes serve as the basis for the clinical advantages seen with NPWT.

INDICATIONS

In addressing purely soft tissue traumatic wounds, the best-supported indication for NPWT is to provide temporary wound cover following thorough debridement when definitive closure is not possible, such as in cases of significant wound contamination, need for subsequent debridement, significant edema, or in a patient who is critically ill. This form of therapy can be quickly applied and accomplishes the goals of prevention of desiccation, minimizing microbial contamination, reduction of edema, and facilitation of wound drainage. Because it is changed less frequently than wet-to-dry dressings and subsequently provides less discomfort for the patient, NPWT is less labor intensive for hospital staff. With regard to indications for its use, NPWT has been particularly successful in the treatment of fasciotomy incisions because delayed primary closure allows for edema to subside and compartment pressures to normalize.[6,7] For similar reasons, NPWT has also been shown to be more effective when applied over surgical wounds or incisions at fracture sites known to have a high incidence of wound complications compared with dry dressings (**Fig. 2**). Several randomized trials in the orthopedic literature support these findings, particularly in high-risk closed extremity and acetabular fractures.[8] In a randomized trial of 263 patients, Stannard and colleagues[9] showed a decreased risk of deep infection and dehiscence in high-risk lower extremity fractures using continuous negative pressure at 125 mm Hg for 2 to 3 days. Animal models have reproduced these findings, showing a mechanism of action through edema reduction, accelerated wound healing, decreased lateral tension on wound edges, and reduction in hematoma or seroma.[10–12]

This therapy has also proved to be a superior means to preserve skin grafts, improve skin graft incorporation, and reepithelialize the donor site. When applied directly over a newly applied skin graft, Llanos and colleagues[13] showed in a randomized trial of 60 subjects that the median rate of skin graft loss and the median hospital stay were significantly reduced compared with a control group.

NPWT has also been successful as a means to downscale the complexity of soft tissue reconstruction (**Fig. 3**). Parrett and colleagues[14] showed a decrease in the number of free flaps needed

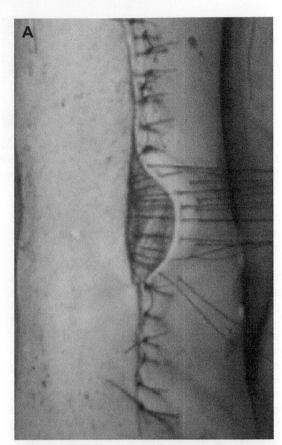

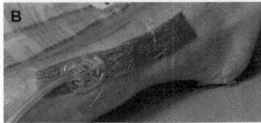

Fig. 2. (*A, B*) The incisional dressing has resulted in decreased rates of infection and other wound complications in patients with total ankle or hip arthroplasty, as well as high-risk incisions after fracture surgery.

when NPWT was used in reconstruction with no difference in infection, nonunion, amputation, or reoperation rates between groups. In progressing a complex wound to a smaller and simpler state, clinicians may avoid morbidity for patients and also reduce cost of care.[15] Although first performing an aggressive debridement of all nonviable soft tissue is advised, NPWT can be a useful tool to promote granulation tissue growth during a state of wound bed unsuitability. Exposed bone, tendon, and orthopedic implants can preclude definitive wound closure. NPWT may enhance tissue granulation over these substrates to allow staged closure.[16–18] However, care must be taken

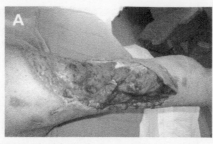
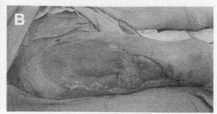

Fig. 3. (*A*) NPWT is ideal for soft tissue defects that can heal through secondary intention or require skin grafting. (*B*) It can serve as an effective way to downscale the complexity of soft tissue reconstruction, as shown after 1 week of NPWT treatment.

to protect any exposed blood vessels or nerves and not place the dressing within too close proximity (**Fig. 4**).

The delivery of negative pressure may also influence its effect on wound healing. These dressings are commonly applied in a continuous negative pressure setting. A standard pressure of −125 mm Hg is applied, based on literature showing a 4-fold increase in blood flow compared with conventional dressings.[19] However, there is more recent support from work performed in a pig model for intermittent or variable pressure application to increase blood flow, wound contraction, and granulation rate.[19,20] These findings have yet to translate into a change of NPWT practice because of a lack of clinical data to corroborate them. In addition, patients find variable and intermittent therapy to be painful, which decreases compliance.

Although the literature is limited, there is evidence to support the use of NPWT in the setting of wound complications when approaching wounds with increased drainage or hematoma (**Fig. 5**). In a prospective randomized study comparing pressure

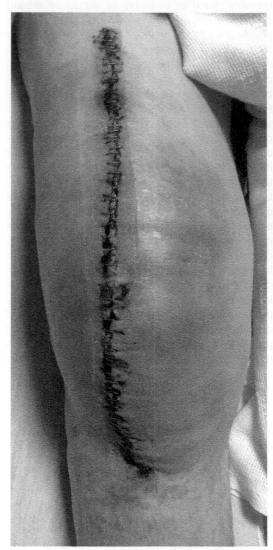

Fig. 5. NPWT can help to manage hematomas and drainage from long wounds, especially in tenuous areas. In this patient, who is status post–revision total knee arthroplasty for periprosthetic fracture, incisional NPWT was placed after hematoma formation in the acute setting. Incisional NPWT is now typically placed as the primary dressing for large wounds and in the obese.

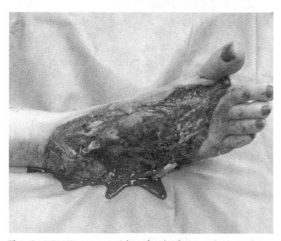

Fig. 4. NPWT can provide a bed of granulation tissue over exposed bone and tendon. However, in tenuous areas, care must be taken to dissect out and protect any exposed blood vessels and/or nerves.

dressings with NPWT in 44 patients, NPWT had continued drainage for approximately half the length of time (1.6 vs 3.1 days) and a decreased infection rate, from 16% to 8%.[21] There is some literature to support NPWT to decrease bacterial load in a contaminated wound.[19] However, more recent literature has refuted this conclusion with mixed findings on its effect on bacterial load.[22–24] Although these dressings can be used to provide provisional coverage of infected wounds, they should not take the place of formal irrigation, debridement, and systemic antibiotics when addressing infection.

COMPLICATIONS AND CHALLENGES

Although infrequent, NPWT is has potential complications and challenges. In the acute setting, careful thought must be applied to the ideal timing of NPWT placement. Although some wounds are ideal for acute, immediate NPWT, others (ie, severe degloving) require a thorough operative debridement and identification of neurovascular structures in order to avoid complications (**Fig. 6**). Other complications, including bleeding, pain during dressing changes, retained sponge with prolonged placement, and wound breakdown, can occur during NPWT. Wound breakdown, particularly in immunocompromised patients, may occur at a higher rate despite NPWT. For example, a 65-year-old, immunocompromised (history of kidney transplant on lifelong immunosuppressants) patient, 8 weeks out from operative fixation of her medial tibial plateau, returned with wound drainage and eventual breakdown despite NPWT (**Fig. 7**A, B). Irrigation, debridement, removal of hardware, and flap coverage were eventually needed (see **Fig. 7**C, D).

However, these complications can be avoided with close monitoring and specific strategies. Avoiding excessive bleeding requires a thorough assessment of the associated wound bed or incision before dressing placement. Following dressing placement, outputs should be monitored closely because the negative pressure environment, particularly in anticoagulated patients, may lead to protracted coagulation and excessive blood loss.[25]

A frequently overlooked complication during NPWT is wound complications secondary to interrupted therapy. Loss of power, or error messages, often arise with a poor seal or with a blockage in the tubing. When this occurs for a prolonged period of time, the negative pressure atmosphere is lost, creating a moist, closed environment that can eventually lead to further skin maceration and breakdown. Cognizant of this potential complication, Collinge and colleagues[26] retrospectively assessed 123 patients who had interrupted NPWT, and reported a significantly increased rate of wound complications compared with patients who did not have interruptions. Thus, all staff must be conscious of prompt notification of any interruptions in therapy, which must be addressed in a timely fashion.

With regard to minimizing pain during dressing changes, some simple principles and strategies can be used. Avoid prolonged days between changes and adhere to the recommended duration of 2 to 4 days. Moistening the interface

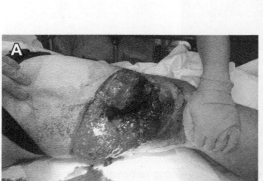
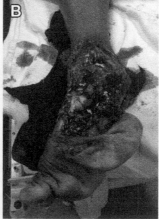

Fig. 6. (A) Certain wounds present as ideal for NPWT, covering a large area of soft tissue without exposed vessels or nerves. (B) Other injuries, such as severe degloving injuries of the lower extremity, often present a different challenge. For these injuries, it is prudent to perform careful and thorough debridement and ensure proper coverage and partial closure combined with strategic NPWT sponge placement a safe distance from nerves and vessels.

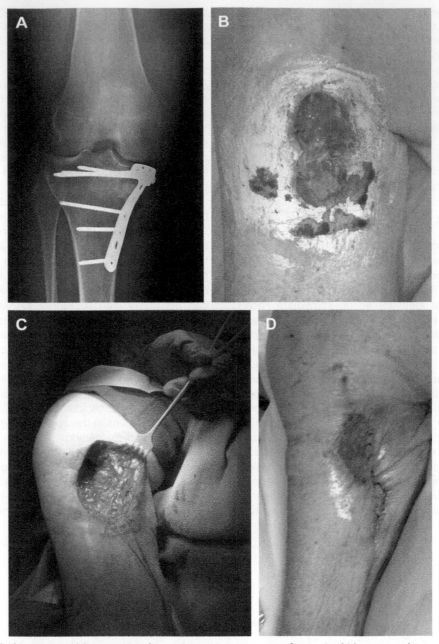

Fig. 7. (*A, B*) This 65-year-old woman on chronic immunosuppressants for a prior kidney transplant returned with drainage, infection, and subsequent dehiscence 8 weeks following operative fixation of her medial tibial plateau. (*C, D*) Despite NPWT, eventual debridement later required flap coverage and skin graft to close the site.

between the sponge and the soft tissue can ease dressing removal. Furthermore, although anecdotally used by the senior authors, application of a nonocclusive protective dressing between the sponge and skin (eg, cellulose acetate silicone dressing, petroleum gauze dressing) can also aid in making dressing removal more facile and prevent irritation or maceration of the skin after prolonged dressing application. Christensen and colleagues[27] performed a prospective, randomized trial comparing the use of topical lidocaine (1%) without epinephrine versus placebo before dressing removal. Patients who received the lidocaine injection directly into the sponge before removal had significantly less pain before removal.[27] Following sponge removal, careful inspection of the wound bed should be performed to avoid leaving behind any free foam material.

SUMMARY

NPWT can be beneficial by optimizing orthopedic wounds and decreasing potential complications. Practical applications include use in open fractures, areas of extensive soft tissue loss, and even primarily closed incisions in high-risk patients. Continuous therapy at 125 mm Hg using the standard large-pore foam sponge is recommended. Outputs should be carefully monitored to avoid excessive bleeding. Pain during dressing changes can be avoided by using a nonadherent barrier between the sponge and the soft tissue, and the use of topical lidocaine can also significantly reduce associated pain. Interruptions in therapy should be avoided and corrected promptly. Although NPWT has advantages, with supportive data, the right indications coupled with diligent ancillary staff education and monitoring are crucial for good outcomes.[26]

REFERENCES

1. Timmers MS, Le Cessie S, Banwell P, et al. The effects of varying degrees of pressure delivered by negative-pressure wound therapy on skin perfusion. Ann Plast Surg 2005;55(6):665–71.

2. Tarkin IS. The versatility of negative pressure wound therapy with reticulated open cell foam for soft tissue management after severe musculoskeletal trauma. J Orthop Trauma 2008;22(10 Suppl):S146–51.

3. Labler L, Rancan M, Mica L, et al. Vacuum-assisted closure therapy increases local interleukin-8 and vascular endothelial growth factor levels in traumatic wounds. J Trauma 2009;66(3):749–57.

4. McNulty AK, Schmidt M, Feeley T, et al. Effects of negative pressure wound therapy on fibroblast viability, chemotactic signaling, and proliferation in a provisional wound (fibrin) matrix. Wound Repair Regen 2007;15(6):838–46.

5. Chen SZ, Cao DY, Li JQ, et al. Effect of vacuum-assisted closure on the expression of proto-oncogenes and its significance during wound healing. Zhonghua Zheng Xing Wai Ke Za Zhi 2005;21(3): 197–200 [in Chinese].

6. Yang CC, Chang DS, Webb LX. Vacuum-assisted closure for fasciotomy wounds following compartment syndrome of the leg. J Surg Orthop Adv 2006;15(1):19–23.

7. Zannis J, Angobaldo J, Marks M, et al. Comparison of fasciotomy wound closures using traditional dressing changes and the vacuum-assisted closure device. Ann Plast Surg 2009;62(4):407–9.

8. Reddix RN Jr, Leng XI, Woodall J, et al. The effect of incisional negative pressure therapy on wound complications after acetabular fracture surgery. J Surg Orthop Adv 2010;19(2):91–7.

9. Stannard JP, Volgas DA, McGwin G 3rd, et al. Incisional negative pressure wound therapy after high-risk lower extremity fractures. J Orthop Trauma 2012;26(1):37–42.

10. Kilpadi DV, Cunningham MR. Evaluation of closed incision management with negative pressure wound therapy (CIM): hematoma/seroma and involvement of the lymphatic system. Wound Repair Regen 2011;19(5):588–96.

11. Meeker J, Weinhold P, Dahners L. Negative pressure therapy on primarily closed wounds improves wound healing parameters at 3 days in a porcine model. J Orthop Trauma 2011;25(12):756–61.

12. Wilkes RP, Kilpad DV, Zhao Y, et al. Closed incision management with negative pressure wound therapy (CIM): biomechanics. Surg Innov 2012;19(1): 67–75.

13. Llanos S, Danilla S, Barraza C, et al. Effectiveness of negative pressure closure in the integration of split thickness skin grafts: a randomized, double-masked, controlled trial. Ann Surg 2006;244(5): 700–5.

14. Parrett BM, Matros E, Pribaz JJ, et al. Lower extremity trauma: trends in the management of soft-tissue reconstruction of open tibia-fibula fractures. Plast Reconstr Surg 2006;117(4):1315–22 [discussion: 1323–4].

15. Herscovici D Jr, Sanders RW, Scaduto JM, et al. Vacuum-assisted wound closure (VAC therapy) for the management of patients with high-energy soft tissue injuries. J Orthop Trauma 2003;17(10): 683–8.

16. Lee HJ, Kim JW, Oh CW, et al. Negative pressure wound therapy for soft tissue injuries around the foot and ankle. J Orthop Surg Res 2009;4:14.

17. Pelham FR, Kubiak EN, Sathappan SS, et al. Topical negative pressure in the treatment of infected wounds with exposed orthopaedic implants. J Wound Care 2006;15(3):111–6.

18. DeFranzo AJ, Argenta LC, Marks MW, et al. The use of vacuum-assisted closure therapy for the treatment of lower-extremity wounds with exposed bone. Plast Reconstr Surg 2001;108(5):1184–91.

19. Morykwas MJ, Argenta LC, Shelton-Brown EI, et al. Vacuum-assisted closure: a new method for wound control and treatment: animal studies and basic foundation. Ann Plast Surg 1997;38(6):553–62.

20. Malmsjo M, Gustafsson L, Lindstedt S, et al. The effects of variable, intermittent, and continuous negative pressure wound therapy, using foam or gauze, on wound contraction, granulation tissue formation, and ingrowth into the wound filler. Eplasty 2012;12:e5.

21. Stannard JP, Robinson JT, Anderson ER, et al. Negative pressure wound therapy to treat hematomas and surgical incisions following high-energy trauma. J Trauma 2006;60(6):1301–6.

22. Moisidis E, Heath T, Boorer C, et al. A prospective, blinded, randomized, controlled clinical trial of topical negative pressure use in skin grafting. Plast Reconstr Surg 2004;114(4):917–22.

23. Weed T, Ratliff C, Drake DB. Quantifying bacterial bioburden during negative pressure wound therapy: does the wound VAC enhance bacterial clearance? Ann Plast Surg 2004;52(3):276–9 [discussion: 279–80].

24. Moues CM, Vos MC, van den Bemd GJ, et al. Bacterial load in relation to vacuum-assisted closure wound therapy: a prospective randomized trial. Wound Repair Regen 2004;12(1):11–7.

25. Li Z, Yu A. Complications of negative pressure wound therapy: a mini review. Wound Repair Regen 2014;22(4):457–61.

26. Collinge C, Reddix R. The incidence of wound complications related to negative pressure wound therapy power outage and interruption of treatment in orthopaedic trauma patients. J Orthop Trauma 2011;25(2):96–100.

27. Christensen TJ, Thorum T, Kubiak EN. Lidocaine analgesia for removal of wound vacuum-assisted closure dressings: a randomized double-blinded placebo-controlled trial. J Orthop Trauma 2013; 27(2):107–12.

Pediatric Orthopaedics

Preface
Pediatric Orthopedics

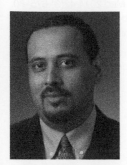

Shital N. Parikh, MD
Editor

Fractures of the distal radius and ulna are one of the most common fractures in children. These fractures must be differentiated from their adult counterparts due to vast differences in their management. Most fractures of the distal radius and ulna in children involve the metaphysis or the physis, and most are treated with closed reduction and immobilization. Many younger children don't even require a closed reduction; for example, in children less than 10 years of age, isolated and overriding fractures of distal radius can be treated with cast immobilization without an attempt at anatomic fracture reduction with satisfactory results.[1] Similarly, physeal fractures of the distal radius in younger children should not be attempted to be reduced after the first 7 to 10 days to prevent physeal injury and resultant growth disturbances; rather they should be allowed to malunite. Radiographic malunion correlates poorly with forearm rotation, and subsequent remodeling should be expected to correct residual deformities.[2] If a closed reduction is required, adequate relaxation and meticulous attention to cast application techniques are necessary. If surgery is indicated, most fractures can be treated with closed reduction and smooth pin fixation. In contrast to distal radius physeal fractures with growth arrest rates of 5 to 7%, similar physeal fractures of distal ulna have a significantly higher growth arrest rate of about 55%.[3] Herman and Pannu provide a comprehensive review of these fractures in children, dividing them based on location and type of fracture and then discussing management principles, including acceptable reduction parameters, nonoperative and operative treatment approaches, and related complications.

There is an apparent increase in pediatric and adolescent sports participation and injuries. A recent study reported on the increasing rate of ACL reconstructions in the skeletally immature over the past 20 years in New York State.[4] There is push from the family and coaches to involve younger and younger children in competitive sports. Such a trend, however, comes with a price. It has long been recognized that there are deleterious physical and psychological effects of competitive sports on the preadolescent child. In 1975, Sayre called attention to the slow and fast maturers, the "drop-out syndrome" in these athletes, and a "ban" on competitive sports involving preadolescent children as a first step toward physical and psychological well-being, that can continue in adulthood.[5] As a physician, it is important to understand the unique skeletal and emotional development in children that differentiates them from an adult. Smucny and colleagues provide a timely review of the short-term and long-term consequences of single-sport specialization in pediatric and adolescent athletes. They provide an overview of the epidemiology of pediatric sports injuries, physiologic and anatomic considerations in young athletes, and tips on assessment of these patients.

Shital N. Parikh, MD
Cincinnati Children's Hospital Medical Center
University of Cincinnati School of Medicine
3333 Burnet Ave
Cincinnati, OH 45229, USA

E-mail address:
Shital.Parikh@cchmc.org

Orthop Clin N Am 46 (2015) xix–xx
http://dx.doi.org/10.1016/j.ocl.2014.12.002
0030-5898/15/$ – see front matter © 2015 Published by Elsevier Inc.

orthopedic.theclinics.com

REFERENCES

1. Crawford SN, Lee LS, Izuka BH. Closed treatment of overriding distal radial fractures without reduction in children. J Bone Joint Surg Am 2012;94(3):246–52.
2. Abzug JM, Little K, Kozin SH. Physeal arrest of the distal radius. J Am Acad Orthop Surg 2014;22(6): 381–9.
3. Golz RJ, Grogan DP, Greene TL, et al. Distal ulnar physeal injury. J Pediatr Orthop 1991;11(3):318–26.
4. Dodwell ER, Lamont LE, Green DW, et al. 20 years of pediatric anterior cruciate ligament reconstruction in New York State. Am J Sports Med 2014;42(3):675–80.
5. Sayre BM. Letter: The need to ban competitive sports involving preadolescent children. Pediatric 1975; 55(4):564–5.

Distal Radius-Ulna Fractures in Children

Gurpal S. Pannu, MD, Marty Herman, MD*

KEYWORDS

- Compartment syndrome • Growth arrest • Arm splint • Displaced fracture

KEY POINTS

- Fractures involving the distal radius-ulna are among the most common fractures seen in the pediatric population.
- Distal radius fractures most often result from a fall onto the outstretched hand. An increasing incidence may be related to trends in leisure/sports activities.
- The vast majority of these fractures may be treated appropriately with closed reduction and casting.
- The clinician should be aware of potential complications such as acute carpal tunnel syndrome, growth arrest and malunion.

INTRODUCTION

Fractures involving the distal radius and ulna are commonly seen in children and adolescents. Management of these injuries in pediatric patients should include assessment of the neurovascular status of the extremity, associated soft-tissue injury, and, most importantly, possible involvement of the physes of the radius and ulna. Treatment of these injuries may vary from simple casting and radiographic follow-up to urgent reduction and surgical fixation. Regardless of the initial treatment plan, the treating surgeon must remain aware of the potential for both early and late complications that may affect outcomes. The clinician often must balance the patient and family's desire for early return to activity with the goal of long-term functionality of the involved limb. Many studies have discussed optimal treatment methods with regards to specific fracture patterns. Nonetheless, management of these injuries tends to differ quite significantly among clinicians. Recently published data have questioned long-held principles of nonoperative management for all fractures. This article reviews distal pediatric forearm fracture management with emphasis on potential complications and discussion related to recently published clinical data.

Epidemiology

Fractures in the pediatric population are common. An annual fracture incidence of 180 per 10,000 in children younger than 16 years has been reported. Fractures of the distal radius were found to be the most common, representing 31% of all fractures in this patient population and tended to occur in the nondominant extremity in roughly 53% of cases. The mean age at the time of fracture was 9.3 years in girls and 10.4 years in boys.[1,2] Pediatric fractures are more commonly seen in boys, with a male to female incidence ratio of 1.5.[2]

Distal radius fractures most often occur as a result of a fall onto the outstretched hand.[3] Randsborg and colleagues[1] reported that activity-related fracture was most common during soccer and the highest fracture rate involved snowboarding. Snowboarding conferred a fracture risk 5 times greater than during trampoline-related activities and 4 times greater than in soccer. Other activities with high fracture risk include handball, rollerblading, and playground activities.

Clinical Evaluation

Initial evaluation of the patient with injury to the wrist and forearm should focus on the soft tissue

Department of Orthopedic Surgery and Pediatrics, Drexel University College of Medicine, 230N Broad Street, Philadelphia, PA 19102, USA
* Corresponding author.
E-mail address: martyj.herman@gmail.com

Orthop Clin N Am 46 (2015) 235–248
http://dx.doi.org/10.1016/j.ocl.2014.11.003
0030-5898/15/$ – see front matter Published by Elsevier Inc.

and neurovascular status. The area of injury must be meticulously inspected for abrasions, lacerations, and the possibility of an open fracture. Although soft-tissue swelling is expected in the setting of musculoskeletal trauma, the clinician should evaluate the forearm compartments and remain vigilant in identifying a developing compartment syndrome. Compartment syndrome in the uncooperative pediatric patient can, at times, be difficult to detect. Cardinal signs of an acute compartment syndrome in a child include an *agitated*, inconsolable child appearing *anxious* and requiring an increasing amount of *analgesia*. This condition can be remembered conveniently as the "Three A's" of pediatric compartment syndrome. Perfusion of the distal extremity may be evaluated by examining radial artery pulse, capillary refill, and temperature of the digits. Neurologic examination consists of inspecting for sensory deficits in the radial, ulnar, and median nerve distributions. Although difficult to assess in a pediatric patient in an acute fracture setting, an attempt should be made to evaluate the anterior interosseus, posterior interosseus, and median and ulnar nerve motor function. The remainder of the involved extremity should be carefully evaluated for concomitant injury, as the patient often may be distracted by their most painful injury.

Plain film imaging of the distal forearm fracture is, in most cases, sufficient for diagnosis and management of distal forearm fractures. It is imperative to obtain adequate anterior-posterior and lateral views of the fracture site. If physical examination reveals pain or decreased range of motion in other sites, additional imaging should be obtained to rule out associated fractures. Computed tomographic (CT) scan and MRI have a limited role in the acute fracture setting but may be useful in the management of chronic sequelae, such as malunion and growth arrest.

NONSURGICAL TREATMENT

Fracture characteristics that may affect treatment include skin integrity, neurovascular status, and fracture displacement. The vast majority of distal radius fractures, however, are closed injuries without neurovascular compromise and are effectively treated with casting alone or closed reduction and cast immobilization.

Metaphyseal Fractures

See **Fig. 1** for 4 different examples of metaphyseal fracture patterns.

Torus fractures
A torus or buckle fracture refers to a unicortical, metaphyseal fracture most often resulting from a fall onto an outstretched hand. The cortex under compression, most commonly the dorsal cortex, fails or buckles, whereas the cortex under tension, most commonly the volar cortex, remains intact. Because of the intact cortex, these fractures are inherently stable. On examination, significant swelling or deformity is usually not seen. Point tenderness on the distal radial metaphysis confirms the diagnosis.

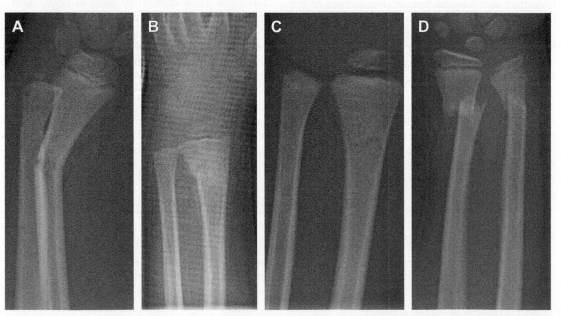

Fig. 1. Distal radius metaphyseal fractures. (*A*) Greenstick fracture, (*B*) buckle fracture, (*C*) complete, nondisplaced fracture, (*D*) complete, displaced fracture.

Torus fractures are treated with a short-arm splint or cast for 3 weeks, and radiographic follow-up of these injuries is typically not necessary.[4,5] Studies have demonstrated that casting may not be necessary to ensure satisfactory healing. The application of a soft bandage or removable splint has been successfully used to treat these injuries.[6–8]

Greenstick fracture

An incomplete fracture involving failure of the tension-sided cortex and plastic deformation of the compression cortex is termed a greenstick fracture. As described by Evans,[9] this injury classically occurs as a result of a compression and rotational deformity. A distal third forearm greenstick fracture most commonly demonstrates an apex volar angulation and represents a supination injury. The reduction maneuver, aiming to counteract the deforming force, involves pronation of the forearm. Alternatively, an apex dorsally angulated fracture, representing a pronation injury, is reduced with supination of the forearm. Correction of the rotational deformity has been shown to be a reliable and easily reproducible reduction maneuver.[10]

Bicortical Fractures

Nondisplaced fractures

Bicortical, or complete, fractures involving the distal radial metaphysis typically result from falls onto an outstretched hand but involve higher energy mechanisms than buckle fractures. Patients with these fractures frequently have associated distal ulna fractures, especially if torsion is combined with axial loading through the outstretched hand. Patients with nondisplaced, bicortical distal radius fractures typically present with pain and swelling about the wrist. On examination, the distal radius is tender to palpation on the metaphysis. For those with associated distal ulna fractures, the metaphysis, styloid, and the triangular fibrocartilage complex (TFCC) may also be painful and tender to touch. Active pronation/supination of the forearm and flexion/extension of the wrist are generally limited secondary to pain. Radiographs reveal a fracture line that extends transversely through the metaphysis.

A well-molded short-arm or-long arm cast is the recommended treatment of these nondisplaced metaphyseal fractures. In the author's experience, patients with nondisplaced fractures of both the radius and ulna and those with painful forearm rotation are more comfortable in a long-arm cast initially. Radiographs should be obtained again at 7 to 10 days after injury to confirm that reduction has been maintained. The cast is removed at 4 to 6 weeks after injury. Adequate healing is confirmed by physical examination and repeat radiographs that show bone healing. After cast removal, instructions are given for range of motion and strengthening exercises; physical therapy is rarely needed. Within 8 to 10 weeks, patients may resume sports and other activities.

Displaced fractures

Patients with displaced fractures of the distal radius metaphysis typically present with a deformity of the wrist. Skin compromise at the fracture site, such as a small laceration or an abrasion with active bleeding, may indicate an open fracture. Neurovascular examination must be documented before reduction is attempted. Because most displaced fractures demonstrate dorsal displacement, the clinician should assess for volar wounds and median nerve injury. Sterile dressing of open wounds and provisional splinting should be done in the emergency department before obtaining radiographs to lessen the risk of ongoing soft-tissue injury and for patient comfort.

Closed reduction Displaced fractures are best treated with closed reduction and immobilization under conscious sedation in the emergency department. Fracture reduction may be facilitated by re-creation of the deformity that would relax the intact periosteum on the compression side of the fracture and allow the distal fracture fragment to slide over the proximal fragment. A well-molded sugar tong splint or cast would help maintain the reduction. When a cast is applied in the acute fracture setting, consideration should be given to bivalve the cast to accommodate subsequent swelling (**Fig. 2**).

After reduction and application of a cast or splint, postreduction radiographs and a repeat clinical examination are mandatory. Most patients may be discharged home with fracture care instructions. Those patients with significant pain, severe swelling, abnormal findings on examination, or a potentially unsuitable home environment are best observed in the hospital overnight. On the hospital floor, instructions are given for strict wrist elevation, frequent neurovascular checks, and pain control that permits reliable evaluation but does not mask the signs of an evolving compartment syndrome or acute carpal tunnel syndrome.

Acute carpal tunnel syndrome, although rare in the pediatric population, has been reported after Salter-Harris (SH) 2 fractures of the distal radius.[11,12] This complication is most common after dorsally angulated and displaced metaphyseal or physeal distal radius fractures in older children and adolescents. Patients developing acute carpal tunnel syndrome initially present with parasthesias in the sensory distribution of the median

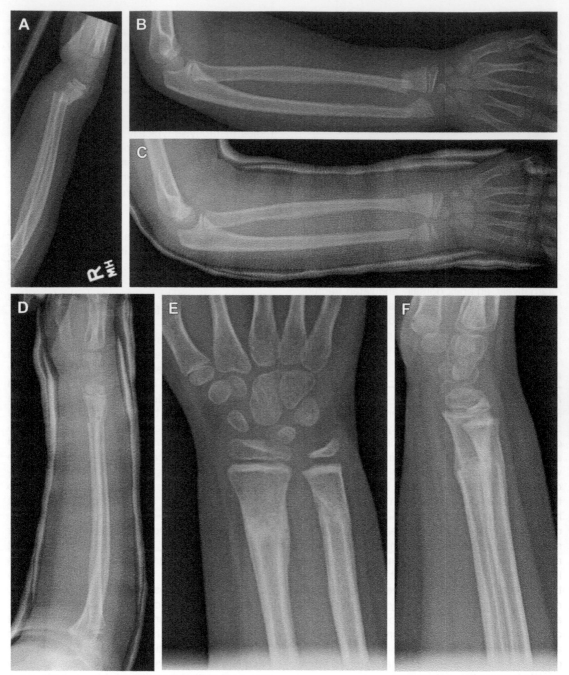

Fig. 2. A 5-year-old girl fell from tricycle and sustained a fracture of the distal radius and ulnar metaphysis with apex volar angulation (*A, B*). The child underwent closed reduction and casting in the emergency room under conscious sedation. Follow-up radiograph at 2 weeks demonstrated a well-maintained reduction (*C, D*). Eight weeks after injury, radiographs reveal a healed fracture in anatomic alignment (*E, F*).

nerve. Differentiating a contusion to the median nerve from acute carpal tunnel syndrome can be challenging. The diagnosis is largely clinical and relies heavily on the progression of symptoms. A median nerve contusion presents as numbness or tingling in the volar aspect of the thumb, index, and long fingers that begins immediately after the injury. The symptoms are nonprogressive and tend to respond to elevation of the extremity and loosening of the dressings. Carpal tunnel syndrome, on the other hand, presents as a gradual progression of symptoms over a few hours after injury. The patient reports no relief with elevation and loosening of dressing.[13] In the setting of progressive median nerve symptoms unrelieved by elevation, an urgent carpal tunnel release is indicated.

Acceptable Reduction of Metaphyseal Fractures

The distal radial physis accounts for 60% of the growth of the radius and typically closes at 14 to 16 years of age. A significant and predictable amount of remodeling occurs in fractures that heal with angulation and displacement if the physis is not injured. Acceptable reduction parameters vary with age (**Table 1**).

Owing to significant degree of remodeling, incomplete reduction of distal radial metaphyseal fractures may yield successful outcomes in children. Crawford and colleagues[14] reported on 51 consecutive patients younger than 10 years with completely displaced distal radius fractures. The fracture was treated with gentle manipulation without sedation or local anesthetics to achieve angulation within 10° of normal. Translation and overriding of the fracture fragments (bayonet opposition) in the sagittal plane was accepted. At follow-up, all patients demonstrated union with full range of motion and radiographic evidence of remodeling. The achievement of a successful outcome without the potential complications and cost of conscious sedation certainly questions the traditional management of these fractures.

Cast considerations

Cast index Several methods to evaluate casting have been developed, all with the purpose of quantifying the characteristics of casting technique that effectively maintains reduction. In the author's opinion, and based on the published literature, the cast index, defined by the distance between inner cast edges measured on the lateral radiograph divided by that measured on the anteroposterior radiograph, is most easily calculated and a reasonable predictor of casting

success.[15,16] Chess and colleagues[17] earlier had demonstrated the importance of the cast index in their study of 558 pediatric patients who underwent casting for forearm and wrist fractures. A significant difference in cast index was noted in those patients who had lost the initial fracture reduction. Webb and colleagues[18] presented 113 patients with distal radius fractures treated with either a long- or short-arm cast. Patients who had failed to maintain the initial reduction had a significantly higher cast index, 0.79, than patients in whom the reduction was maintained, 0.71.

Short-arm versus long-arm casting Controversy exists regarding the optimal length of the cast that best maintains reduction of displaced fractures. Traditionally, long-arm casts have been used after reduction of displaced distal radius. It was thought that this enhanced maintenance of reduction because elbow motion, more specifically pronation and supination, was restricted. Studies have shown, however, that short-arm casting may be equally efficacious in maintaining reduction. The quality of reduction and cast molding are more important factors in the prevention of late displacement than the length of the cast. Advocates of short-arm casting also demonstrated an advantage for patients, documenting that patients treated with below-elbow casts missed fewer days of school and required less assistance with activities of daily living than patients in long-arm casts.[19]

Outpatient follow-up Regardless of the length of cast or quality of reduction, late fracture displacement is common. Approximately a third of displaced distal radius fractures lose reduction, emphasizing the importance of close radiographic follow-up.[20,21] Several factors may increase the risk of late displacement, including initial displacement (>50% translation, >30° angulation, bayonet apposition), incomplete reduction, concomitant distal ulna fracture, and poor casting technique. Weekly clinical and radiographic follow-up for 2 to 3 weeks after reduction is recommended to ensure that displacement is identified before fracture healing with malunion. Repeat closed fracture reduction of metaphyseal fractures may be safe for up to 2 to 3 weeks from injury. For most fractures, cast immobilization is used for a total of 4 to 6 weeks. Return to full activities can be expected at 2 to 3 months after injury, depending on the age of the child.

Physeal Fractures of the Distal Radius

Fractures of the distal radial physis are among the most common growth plate injuries seen in the pediatric population. Most of these injuries are SH 1 and 2 fractures (**Table 2**).[22] The risk of growth

Table 1
Acceptable residual angulation after fracture of the distal radius

Age (y)	Sagittal Plane (°)	Coronal Plane (°)
4–9	15–20	15
9–11	10–15	5
11–13	10	0
>13	0–5	0

Adapted from Rockwood CA, Beaty JH, Kasser JR. Rockwood and Wilkins' fractures in children. 7th edition. Lippincott Williams and Wilkins; 2010; with permission.

Table 2
Salter-Harris fractures of distal radius

Salter-Harris 1	22%
Salter-Harris 2	58%
Salter-Harris 3	2.6%
Salter-Harris 4	2.0%
Salter-Harris 5	0.4%

Adapted from Lee BS, Esterhai JL Jr, Das M. Fracture of the distal radial epiphysis: characteristics and surgical treatment of premature, post-traumatic epiphyseal closure. Clin Orthop Relat Res 1984;185:90–6; with permission.

arrest after distal radius physeal fracture is about 4%. Although rare, it is the possibility of growth disturbance that sets these fractures apart from metaphyseal fractures.[23] Although the short-term management of these fractures mirrors closely that of metaphyseal fractures, important differences must be noted.

Nondisplaced fractures

Nondisplaced or minimally displaced fractures of the distal radial physis are common. The patient typically complains of wrist pain after a fall onto an outstretched hand without deformity or significant swelling. The examination is notable only for point tenderness on the distal radial physis. Radiographs may reveal a nondisplaced or minimally displaced fracture, most commonly SH 1 or 2 fractures. These fractures are treated with 3 to 4 weeks of immobilization similar to a torus or buckle fracture of the metaphysis. Often, however, radiographs show normal findings. In this scenario, it is the author's practice to diagnose these injuries as occult SH 1 fractures. These injuries are often confused with wrist sprain or contusion. Owing to pain with activities and risk of a subsequent injury that can lead to displacement, these injuries are treated with cast immobilization.

Displaced fractures

Closed reduction SH 1 and 2 fractures constitute the vast majority of displaced distal radius physeal fractures. Although closed reduction under conscious sedation in the emergency department is the best method of initial treatment, the surgeon must be careful to avoid excessive forceful or aggressive maneuvers for reduction, emphasizing instead the use of longitudinal traction and gentle repositioning to limit shear forces across the physis. Multiple attempts at reduction should also be avoided. Finally, because physeal healing is more rapid than healing of metaphyseal fractures, attempts at closed reduction of displaced SH 1 and 2 fractures later than 7 to 10 days after

initial injury are not recommended. Not only is it likely that realignment will not be achieved, late reduction attempts increase the risk of iatrogenic physeal injury and growth arrest. Owing to the tremendous remodeling potential of these injuries, observation of deformity for remodeling is preferred over improving alignment at the risk of injuring the physis.

Owing to rapid healing of physeal fractures compared with metaphyseal fractures, repeat clinical examination and radiographs within 5 to 7 days of injury are recommended to ensure that loss of alignment is identified in such time that safe repeat closed reduction can be performed. Cast immobilization is maintained for around 4 weeks. By then, healing of distal radial physeal fractures is typically complete, as evidenced by resolution of point tenderness and radiographic healing. After cast removal, a removable splint may be applied and instructions for home exercises are given. Full return to activities can be expected within 8 to 12 weeks after injury. Because of the risk of growth arrest, patients should be followed up with radiographs at 6 monthly intervals till growth is documented or till skeletal maturity.

Salter-Harris 3 and 4 Fractures

SH 3 and 4 fractures are rare, occurring predominantly in older patients and in those with high-energy injuries associated with axial loading of the distal radius. At times, plain radiographs alone may not permit adequate assessment of the fracture pattern and displacement. In these cases, CT evaluation may be necessary. Nondisplaced fractures are treated similar to nondisplaced SH 1 and 2 fractures. Displaced fractures require special attention. Because these fractures are intraarticular and involve the physis, achieving anatomic or near-anatomic alignment is essential to improve the chances of successful outcomes. In some cases closed reduction and casting may achieve reduction, whereas most cases require percutaneous manipulation and pinning or open reduction and fixation.

Distal Ulna Fractures

Metaphyseal fractures

Distal ulnar metaphyseal fractures occur most commonly in the setting of an ipsilateral distal radius fracture after a fall from height onto an outstretched hand. Most distal ulna fractures achieve reduction indirectly during reduction of the distal radius fractures. Complete displacement with bayonet apposition and angulation of 20° to 30° are acceptable if the parameters of the radial reduction are within the accepted limits of remodeling. In rare cases, percutaneous reduction and pinning or open reduction are indicated for distal ulna fractures with unacceptable alignment. Healing of distal ulna metaphyseal is achieved in most cases by the cast immobilization used to treat the radius fracture.

Ulnar styloid and distal ulnar physeal fractures

SH fractures of the distal ulna are uncommon. SH 1 and 2 fractures most commonly occur in combination with distal radius fractures. As with metaphyseal ulna fractures, reduction of displaced fractures frequently occurs passively with reduction of the radius fracture and heal uneventfully. Clinical and radiographic follow-up of these fractures is important because of the risk of growth arrest resulting in ulnar shortening, a potentially problematic complication of these injuries. Growth arrest of the distal ulna has been reported to occur in 55% of physeal injuries, a figure dramatically higher than that seen in the distal radius.[24]

In most cases, fractures of the ulnar styloid occur in the setting of fractures of the distal radius in children and adolescents. Cast immobilization used to treat the radius fractures leads to healing of some ulnar styloid fractures, but most do not unite radiographically. Despite nonunion, the vast majority of patients demonstrate excellent clinical outcomes without complaints of ulnar-sided wrist pain, instability, or functional limitation[25] because in most cases, the TFCC remains intact and distal radioulnar joint (DRUJ) stability is not compromised. Symptomatic nonunion of the ulnar styloid presents with painful clicking and ulnar-sided wrist pain. This condition is best treated with excision of the nonunion and fixation of the TFCC to the base of the ulnar styloid.[23] The rare fracture through the base of the ulnar styloid, often a result of high-energy trauma, is associated with DRUJ instability. When such a fracture is identified, some researchers recommend treatment with tension-band fixation and TFCC repair.[23]

Pediatric Galeazzi fracture

Distal radius fractures with associated DRUJ disruption, commonly termed Galeazzi fractures, are most often the result of axial loading of the wrist with extreme pronation. In the pediatric patient, DRUJ instability is most commonly a result of a displaced distal ulnar physeal injury (Fig. 3). Unlike in adults, the ligaments that stabilize the DRUJ remain intact and are attached to the ulnar epiphyseal fracture fragment. Because of this, the vast majority of Galeazzi fractures in children may be managed successfully with closed

reduction and cast immobilization, with the forearm in supination. Surgical intervention is reserved for irreducible DRUJ disruption, which most commonly occurs secondary to extensor carpi ulnaris tendon or periosteal interposition. Potential long-term sequelae of these injuries include limitations of supination and pronation, ulnar nerve dysfunction, and persistent DRUJ instability.

SURGICAL MANAGEMENT
Indications for Surgery

Most displaced fractures of the distal radius are treated with closed reduction and cast immobilization. Surgical treatment is indicated for open fractures, floating elbow, fractures that cannot be adequately reduced with closed reduction, and fractures that have lost reduction.

Zamzam and Khoshhal[21] recommended that completely displaced distal radius fractures be reduced and pinned primarily, citing the high rates of failure when closed reduction and casting was attempted. It was previously suggested that fractures demonstrating initial translation of more than 50% undergo primary fixation.[26] Other studies that have compared closed reduction and casting with percutaneous pinning have reported equivalent clinical outcomes.[20,27] Miller and colleagues[20] found that, although loss of reduction was reported in 39% nonoperative patients, 38% of surgically treated patients had pin-related complications such as pin tract infections and superficial radial sensory nerve irritation. Despite the possible complications of closed reduction and casting and the potential for loss of reduction, it is the author's opinion that primary pinning of all displaced pediatric distal radius fractures is not recommended.

Open Fractures

Initial treatment of open fractures includes administration of intravenous antibiotics, the most important factor in prevention of infection (Box 1). The fracture is then closed reduced under sedation, a sterile dressing is applied to the wound, and a cast or splint is applied. The timing for operative irrigation and debridement is controversial, but all open fractures are best treated with irrigation and debridement in the operating room at the earliest. In pediatric patients, it has been shown that infection rates are similar for patients who have surgery less than 6 to 8 hours after injury compared with those who had surgery between 8 and 24 hours after injury, as long as antibiotics are given in the emergency department.[28]

In the operating room, the open wound is extended to permit inspection of the bone ends,

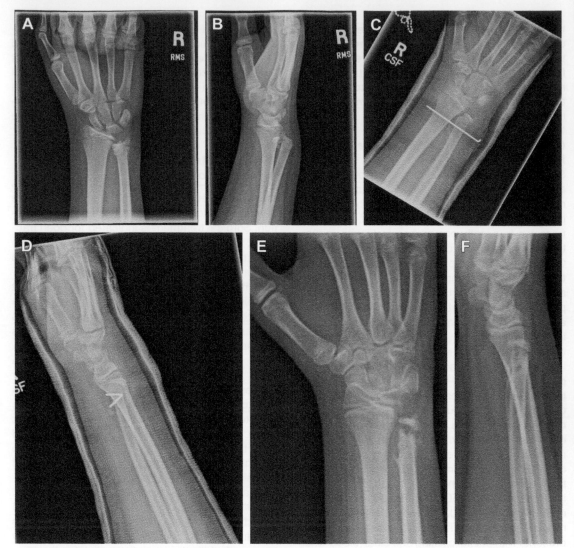

Fig. 3. Galeazzi injury: A 10-year-old boy fell off of a skateboard and sustained a Salter-Harris 4 fracture of the distal ulnar physis along with disruption of the DRUJ (*A, B*). The patient subsequently underwent pinning of the DRUJ (*C, D*). Radiographs at 3-month follow-up (*E, F*).

Box 1
Open fracture protocol

1. Antibiotic administration

   a. Intravenous (IV) Ancef 25 mg/kg (continue every 8 hours)

   b. If type 3, add IV gentamicin 4 mg/kg (once daily)

   c. If farm injury or soiled wound, add penicillin

   d. Duration: 24 to 48 hours, or until final wound closure

2. Confirm tetanus status

3. Irrigation and debridement within 24 hours

4. Wound surveillance

---

removal of debris and nonviable tissue, and thorough irrigation. Depending on the extent and quality of the soft tissue, the wound may be closed primarily or negative-pressure wound therapy may be used. Repeat operative debridement may be necessary. In most cases, the fracture is stabilized with fixation and splinted. After irrigation and debridement, intravenous antibiotics are administered for 24 to 48 hours before discharge.

Closed Reduction and Pinning

Closed reduction and percutaneous pinning is an effective method to maintain satisfactory alignment of the unstable distal radius fracture. Although some metaphyseal or metadiaphyseal fractures are stabilized by a pin proximal to the physis, most metaphyseal fractures are stabilized with a smooth K-wire that crosses the physis. For some fractures, engagement of the distal fragment with the wire may allow the surgeon to use it in a joystick fashion to aid in reduction. An alternative is the use of intrafocal pinning. A pin is introduced at the fracture site, and engagement of the proximal fragment allows correction of the deformity through levering of the distal fragment. This technique may be beneficial in the treatment of difficult fractures with significant preoperative deformity and a distal location rendering conventional pinning difficult. There is also the added benefit of sparing the physis from pinning. Parikh and colleagues[29] demonstrated the efficacy of intrafocal pinning and noted a complication rate no higher than that seen with conventional pinning.

After pinning, a short- or long-arm cast is applied. At the author's institution, patients are not discharged home with oral antibiotics. The pin is generally removed in the office 3 to 4 weeks after surgery, once initial radiographic healing is obtained (**Fig. 4**).

Several studies have reported that pin tract infection after closed reduction and percutaneous pinning are rare and, when present, tend to be superficial in nature.[20,26,30] Superficial infections generally respond well to pin-site care and oral antibiotics and rarely require operative management. Tosti and colleagues[31] reviewed 17 years of data from a single institution and found 12 serious infections related to smooth pins in 884 cases (1.4%) that required hospitalization or reoperation. Diagnoses included cellulitis, osteomyelitis, septic arthritis, and soft-tissue abscess. The presentation ranged from postoperative day 7 to 78, reflecting the importance of remaining vigilant in identification of infection after pinning. It is important to recognize possible pin-tract infection early to decrease the risk of progression to deeper soft-tissue abscess or osteomyelitis.

Open Reduction and Internal Fixation

The most common indications for open reduction include open fractures, irreducible fractures after attempted closed reduction, malunited fractures that are incompletely healed and require osteoclasis to achieve reduction, and intraarticular fractures. Although plate fixation is an option, pin fixation is more commonly used to stabilize fractures after open reduction. Open reduction and plate fixation is indicated for severely comminuted fractures, intraarticular fractures such as SH 3 and 4 fractures, and certain fractures at the metaphyseal-diaphyseal junction that are not amenable to percutaneous pinning because of an extreme pin trajectory (**Fig. 5**).

Dorsal approach
Irreducible or incompletely healed metaphyseal fractures that cannot be closed reduced are best treated with a limited dorsal approach and percutaneous pin fixation. A 2- to 3-cm dorsal wrist incision is made in line with the ulnar border of the brachioradialis tendon centered at the fracture site. The extensor retinaculum is divided, and the interval between the brachioradialis and the extensor tendons is divided and the fracture site exposed dorsally. Using a freer-elevator or a small periosteal elevator, the fracture is gently manipulated to remove interposed tissue and break up early callus. Open reduction is then performed and confirmed with fluoroscopy. The fracture is then pinned as described for closed reduction and percutaneous fixation.

SH 3 and 4 fractures with unacceptable intraarticular alignment are best treated with open reduction regardless of the timing of presentation and may require a more extensile exposure to achieve reduction and place fixation.

Volar approach
Open reduction through a volar approach is most commonly used for apex volar angulated fractures, especially those with intraarticular extension. When plate fixation is necessary, such as for comminuted fractures, it is the author's preference to place fixation on the volar distal radius, as opposed to the dorsal surface. Although plate fixation may be used for metaphyseal fractures in any age, plates that cross the physis are only appropriate for adolescents with less than 2 years of growth remaining.

ACUTE CARPAL TUNNEL SYNDROME
Growth Arrest and Malunion

Growth arrest after fracture involving the distal radius physis is rare, occurring in approximately 4% to 5% of cases.[23] The patient and family should be informed of this risk. Published reports have demonstrated instances of distal radius growth arrest after a metaphyseal fracture not clearly involving the physis. This condition, however, is rare and likely represents an SH 5 crush injury to the physis, a diagnosis that can only be made in retrospect.[32] Patients with a distal radius physeal arrest present early on with only radiographic evidence of abnormal physeal growth manifested by a change in the alignment of the distal radius or relative shortening of the radius compared with the ulna (positive ulnar variance). As deformity worsens with growth, patients note prominence of the ulna and often develop ulnar-sided wrist pain with activities and limited motion. Surgical intervention is indicated with the goals of restoring neutral ulnar variance, a competent DRUJ, and a

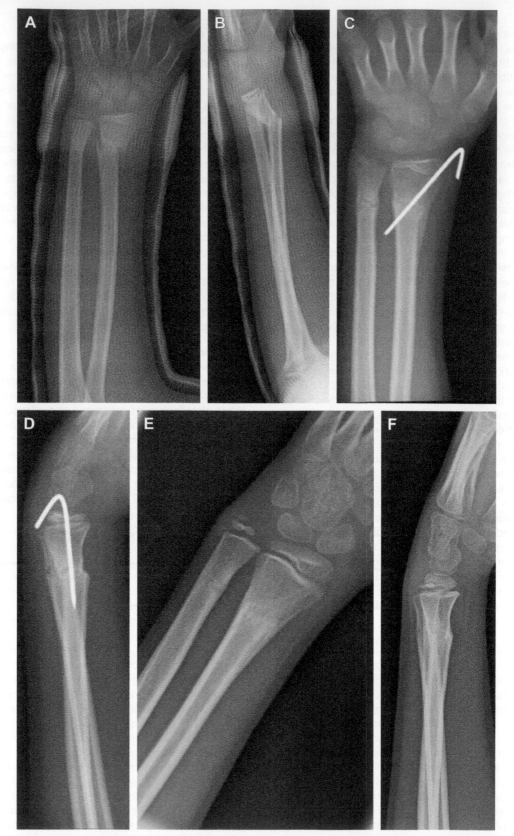

Fig. 4. A 10-year-old girl with a translated and volarly angulated distal radius fracture (*A*, *B*). The patient was treated with closed reduction and percutaneous pinning (*C*, *D*). The fracture healed without residual deformity (*E*, *F*).

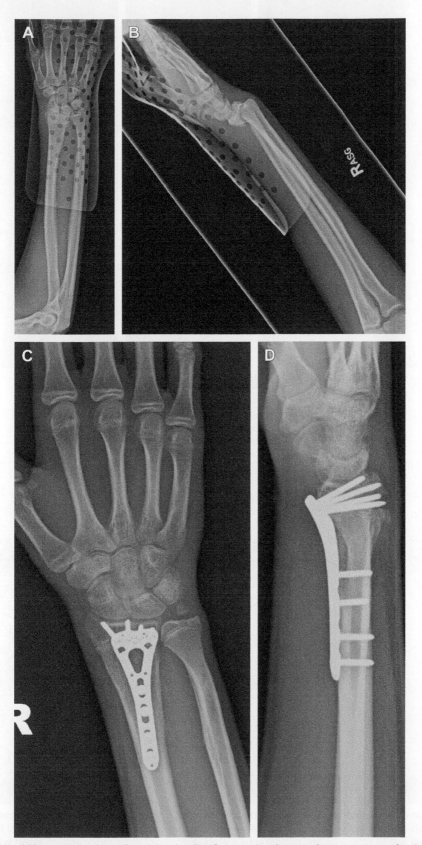

Fig. 5. A 16-year-old boy sustained angulated distal radius fracture (*A*, *B*). He underwent open reduction internal fixation with a volar plate (*C*, *D*). Because he was nearly skeletally mature, the surgeon chose to cross the growth plate.

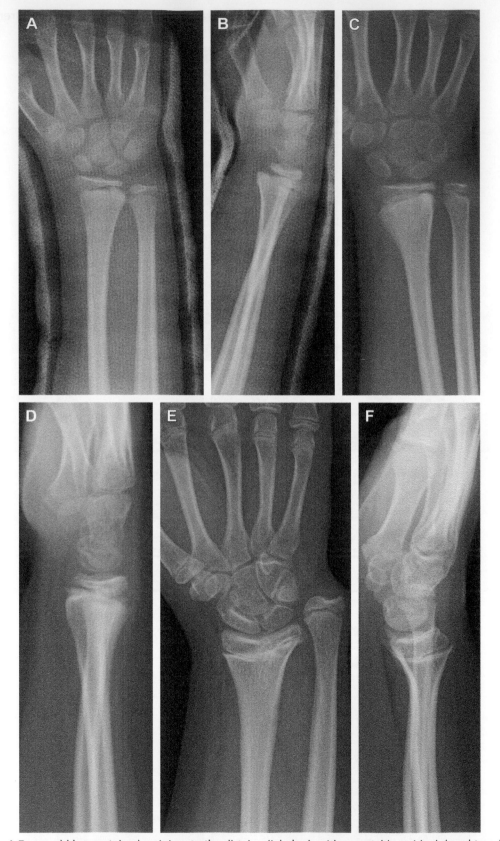

Fig. 6. A 7-year-old boy sustained an injury to the distal radial physis with acceptable residual dorsal translation of the epiphysis after reduction (*A, B*). At 5 weeks follow-up, radiographs demonstrated a healed fracture (*C, D*). The patient was lost to follow-up and radiographs 3 years later depict distal radial growth arrest with a markedly positive ulnar variance (*E, F*). The patient underwent an ulnar shortening osteotomy and epiphysiodesis, along with ulnar-sided radial hemiephysiodesis (*G, H*).

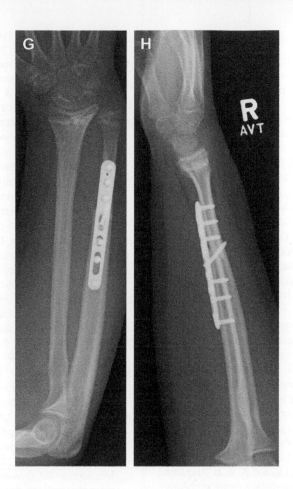

Fig. 6. (*continued*)

nonpainful TFCC. For patients with minimal deformity and at least 2 years of growth remaining, bar resection and local fat interposition may be attempted. Identification of the exact location of the bar is critical and is most reliably accomplished with MRI.[33] For complete radial arrest without deformity, ulnar shortening osteotomy with possible distal ulnar epiphyseodesis is the best option (**Fig. 6**). Concomitant wrist arthroscopy may be necessary if TFCC pathology is suspected. For more complex deformities that result from growth arrest of the distal radius, a combination of radial osteotomy and lengthening with ulnar-sided surgery may be indicated.

The risk of malunion after a distal radius fracture is rare given the remodeling potential of the pediatric patient. However, in the symptomatic patient with significant deformity in a healed fracture, a distal radius corrective osteotomy is indicated. An attempt is made to restore volar tilt and at least 10° of radial inclination with the overall goal of restoring alignment, improving motion, and decreasing the risk of subsequent secondary carpal arthritis and instability.[34]

SUMMARY

Metaphyseal and physeal fractures of the distal radius in children are common. Most cases are best treated with closed reduction and cast immobilization. Although some aspects of care differ among clinicians, long-term outcomes of these injuries are uniformly excellent when specific treatment principles of reduction and casting are followed. Surgical indications are limited and include open fractures, intraarticular fractures, irreducible fractures, and unstable fractures demonstrating late displacement. Closed reduction and percutaneous pin fixation is most commonly used for surgical management, but open reduction and plate fixation is occasionally used, especially for adolescents with intraarticular fractures. The clinician should be aware of the most important complications of distal radius fractures, including infection, acute carpal tunnel syndrome, and growth disturbance of the distal radius, and understand the management of these problems to ensure successful long-term outcomes.

REFERENCES

1. Randsborg PH, Gulbrandsen P, Benth JS, et al. Fractures in children: epidemiology and activity-specific fracture rates. J Bone Joint Surg Am 2013; 95:e42 (1–4).

2. Hedstrom EM, Svensson O, Bergstrom U, et al. Epidemiology of fractures in children and adolescents. Acta Orthop 2010;81(1):148–53.

3. Rodriguez-Merchan EC. Pediatric fractures of the forearm. Clin Orthop Relat Res 2005;432:65–72.

4. Davidson JS, Brown DJ, Barnes SN, et al. Simple treatment for torus fractures of the distal radius. J Bone Joint Surg Br 2001;83B:1173–5.

5. Solan MC, Rees R, Daly K. Current management of torus fractures of the distal radius. Injury 2002;33:503–5.

6. Vernooij CM, Vreeburg ME, Segers MJ, et al. Treatment of torus fractures in the forearm in children using bandage therapy. J Trauma Acute Care Surg 2012;72:1093–7.

7. Kropman RHJ, Bemelman M, Segers MJM, et al. Treatment of impacted greenstick forearm fractures in children using bandage or cast therapy: a prospective randomized trial. J Trauma 2010;68:425–8.

8. West S, Andrews J, Bebbington A, et al. Buckle fractures of the distal radius are safely treated in a soft bandage: a randomized prospective trial of bandage versus plaster cast. J Pediatr Orthop 2005;25:322–5.

9. Evans EM. Fractures of the radius and ulna. J Bone Joint Surg Br 1951;33B:548–61.

10. Tongel AV, Ackerman P, Liekens K, et al. Angulated greenstick fractures of the distal forearm in children: closed reduction by pronation or supination. Acta Orthop Belg 2011;77(l):21–6.

11. Sterling P, Haberman ET. Acute post traumatic median nerve compression associated with Salter II fracture dislocation of the wrist. Bull Hosp Joint Dis 1963;34:167.

12. Binfield PM, Scott-Miknas A, Good CJ. Median nerve compression associated with displaced Salter-Harris type II radial epiphyseal fracture. Injury 1998;29(2):93–4.

13. Schnetzler KA. Acute carpal tunnel syndrome. J Am Acad Orthop Surg 2008;16(5):276–82.

14. Crawford SN, Lee LS, Izuka BH. Closed treatment of overriding distal radial fractures without reduction in children. J Bone Joint Surg Am 2012;94(3):246–52.

15. Debnath UK, Guha AR, Das S. Distal forearm fractures in children: cast index as predictor of re-manipulation. Indian J Orthop 2011;45(4):341–6.

16. McQuinn AG, Jaarsma RL. Risk factors for redisplacement of pediatric distal forearm and distal radius fractures. J Pediatr Orthop 2012;32:687–92.

17. Chess DG, Hyndman JC, Leahey JL, et al. Short arm plaster cast for distal pediatric forearm fractures. J Pediatr Orthop 1994;14:211–3.

18. Webb GR, Galpin RD, Armstrong DG. Comparison of short and long arm plaster casts for displaced fractures in the distal third of the forearm in children. J Bone Joint Surg Am 2006;88A:9–17.

19. Bohm ER, Bubbar V, Yong Hing K, et al. Above and below-the-elbow plaster casts for distal forearm fractures in children. A randomized controlled trial. J Bone Joint Surg Am 2006;88A:1–8.

20. Miller BS, Taylor B, Widmann RF, et al. Cast immobilization versus percutaneous pin fixation of displaced distal radius fractures in children: a prospective, randomized study. J Pediatr Orthop 2005;25:490–4.

21. Zamzam MM, Khoshhal KI. Displaced fracture of the distal radius in children: factors responsible for re-displacement after closed reduction. J Bone Joint Surg Br 2005;87B:841–3.

22. Lee BS, Esterhai JL Jr, Das M. Fracture of the distal radial epiphysis: characteristics and surgical treatment of premature, post-traumatic epiphyseal closure. Clin Orthop Relat Res 1984;185:90–6.

23. Rockwood CA, Beaty JH, Kasser JR. Rockwood and Wilkins' fractures in children. 7th edition. Lippincott Williams and Wilkins; 2010.

24. Golz RJ, Grogan DP, Greene TL, et al. Distal ulnar physeal injury. J Pediatr Orthop 1991;11:318–26.

25. Abid A, Accadbled F, Kany J, et al. Ulnar styloid fractures in children: a retrospective study of 46 cases. J Pediatr Orthop B 2008;17:15–9.

26. Choi KY, Chan WS, Lam TP, et al. Percutaneous Kirschner-wire pinning for severely displaced distal radius fractures in children. A report of 157 cases. J Bone Joint Surg Br 1995;77(5):797–801.

27. McLauchlan GJ, Cowan B, Annan IH, et al. Management of completely displaced metaphyseal fractures of the distal radius in children: a prospective, randomized controlled trial. J Bone Joint Surg Br 2002;84B:413–7.

28. Skaggs DL, Friend L, Alman B, et al. The effect of surgical delay on acute infection following 554 open fractures in children. J Bone Joint Surg Am 2005;87(1):8–12.

29. Parikh S, Jain V, Youngquist J. Intrafocal pinning for distal radius metaphyseal fractures in children. Orthopedics 2013;36:783–8.

30. Hsu LP, Schwartz EG, Kalainov DM, et al. Complications of K-wire fixation in procedures involving wrist and hand. J Hand Surg Am 2011;36(4):610–6.

31. Tosti R, Foroohar A, Pizzutillo PD, et al. Kirschner wire infections in pediatric orthopaedic surgery: a 17-year experience. J Pediatr Orthop 2014;29. [Epub ahead of print].

32. Tang CW, Kay RM, Skaggs DL. Growth arrest of the distal radius following a metaphyseal fracture: case report and review of the literature. J Pediatr Orthop B 2002;11(1):89–92.

33. Azbug JM, Little K, Kozin SH. Physeal arrest of the distal radius. J Am Acad Orthop Surg 2014;22(6):381.

34. Waters PM, Bae DS, Montgomery KD. Surgical management of posttraumatic distal radial growth arrest in adolescents. J Pediatr Orthop 2002;22(6):717–24.

Consequences of Single Sport Specialization in the Pediatric and Adolescent Athlete

Mia Smucny, MD[a], Shital N. Parikh, MD[b],
Nirav K. Pandya, MD[c],*

KEYWORDS

- Pediatric • Adolescent • Sports injuries • Specialization • Burnout • Youth • Overuse

KEY POINTS

- An increasing number of youth are specializing in single sports at younger ages and engaging in repetitive, intensive activity.
- Early, single sport specialization has not been shown to improve future athletic performance, but has been shown to be detrimental both physically and emotionally.
- The adolescent growth spurt is a particularly vulnerable period of time for the youth athlete with repetitive microtrauma, placing the body at risk structurally.
- Identifying burnout is critical for the clinician taking care of youth athletes who specialize in a single sport.
- Long-term consequences extending into adulthood exist for the athlete who specializes at a young age.

EPIDEMIOLOGY OF YOUTH SPORTS PARTICIPATION

Organized sports participation among young athletes has increased tremendously over the past several years. According to the National Council on Youth Sports, nearly 60 million youth between the ages of 6 to 18 participated in organized athletics in 2008 compared with 52 million in 2000.[1] This rise has occurred with a concurrent drop in school-based physical education, with only 29% of all high school students participating in daily classes.[2] This has created an environment in which sports activity is highly structured and centered on the development of specific skills (eg, pitching, tumbling, dribbling) rather than a strong foundation centered around core physical principles, such as flexibility, endurance, and balance. This trend from unstructured free play to deliberate, adult activity has been well-documented in the media,[3,4] and has occurred simultaneously with youth sports becoming a profitable business entity.[5,6]

As a result, a culture has been created in which the definition of success in youth sports is defined not by laying the foundation for a healthy lifestyle, but rather the attainment of "elite" status. This

The authors have no conflicts of interest to disclose.
[a] Department of Orthopaedic Surgery, University of California San Francisco, 500 Parnassus Avenue, MU-320W, San Francisco, San Francisco, CA 94143, USA; [b] Department of Orthopaedic Surgery, Cincinnati Children's Hospital, 3333 Burnet Avenue, Cincinnati, OH 45229, USA; [c] Department of Orthopaedic Surgery, University of California San Francisco Benioff Children's Hospital Oakland, 747 52nd Street, Oakland, CA 94609, USA
* Corresponding author. Department of Pediatric Orthopaedic Surgery, University of California San Francisco Benioff Children's Hospital Oakland, 747 52nd Street, Oakland, CA 94609.
E-mail address: PandyaN@orthosurg.ucsf.edu

Orthop Clin N Am 46 (2015) 249–258
http://dx.doi.org/10.1016/j.ocl.2014.11.004
0030-5898/15/$ – see front matter © 2015 Elsevier Inc. All rights reserved.

push has been largely created by coaches and parents, many of whom measure their child's athletic participation by the attainment of collegiate scholarships and professional contracts. In 1993, Ericsson and colleagues[7] proposed that, to achieve expertise as a musician, one must practice 10,000 hours within that specialized field. This principle has been adopted by many parents as a justification for intensive, adult-style training for sports at increasingly younger ages. As a result, rather than playing a wide variety of sports at a moderate level of intensity during the early stages of physical development, there is increasing evidence that children are beginning to specialize at younger ages in 1 sport.[8–11] This trend is occurring even with multiple groups advocating delayed specialization.[12–15]

Single sport specialization can be defined as intensive, year-round training in a single sport at the exclusion of other sports.[16,17] This phenomenon is especially present in the media, whose attention is focused on athletic prodigies such as Tiger Woods, who are applauded for their dedication to a single sport as toddlers, rather than athletes, such as Steve Nash and Roger Federer, who have achieved similar levels of success while playing multiple sports in their youth.[4] Unfortunately, the desire to specialize is fallacious on multiple fronts.

First, the probability of achieving elite status is small for the vast majority of athletes. According to data published by the National Collegiate Athletic Association in 2013, the estimated probability of competing in collegiate athletics for high school athletes ranged from 3.3% to 6.8% for men's basketball, women's basketball, football, baseball, and men's soccer.[18] For that same group of sports, the estimated probability of competing at the professional level for high school athletes ranged from 0.03% to 0.5%.[18] When these data are coupled with the fact that the average athletic scholarship is approximately $10,000,[19] there is clearly a disconnect between the realistic chances of playing at the next level and, if one does make it, the rather modest amount of money that will be obtained. However, the argument could be made by some that, although the proposed rewards of single sport specialization are difficult to obtain, there exists either no other means to achieve that goal and/or the negative effects of attempting to achieve that path are minimal. The literature suggests otherwise.

From a theoretic perspective, Abernathy et al[20] have suggested that diversified sport training in early and middle adolescence may better foster elite athletic potential than specialization owing to a more positive transfer of skills. Looking at the youngest of cohorts, Fransen and colleagues[21] analyzed 735 boys aged 10 to 12 years of age and found that those who participated in various sports performed better on a standing broad jump and gross motor coordination than those who specialized in a single sport. Gullich and Emrich[22,23] examined athletic performance in Germany and found that the younger the age of recruitment of the athlete into specialized training programs, the earlier they left sports. Those athletes who progressed to higher levels of participation began playing sports at later ages.

At the collegiate level, DiFiori[24] examined a cohort of Division I athletes at their institution and found that 88% had participated in 2 to 3 sports as children, with the vast majority (70%) not specializing until the age of 12. In addition, the average age of specialization between collegiate athletes (15.4 years) and noncollegiate athletes (14.2 years) varied significantly.[24] Malina[17] also found that, among female collegiate athletes in the United States (particularly diving, tennis, golf, track and field, basketball, and volleyball), the majority had their first organized sporting experience in another sport. In addition, Vaeyens and colleagues[25] found that an early age of onset of high-volume, sport-specific training did not necessarily associate with success at the international level in adult sporting activity. Thus, the proposed benefits of single sport specialization are minimal.

In addition, there are multiple studies that document the overall negative effects of sports specialization in the context of limited future gain. Jayanthi and colleagues[26] examined more than 1200 athletes between the ages of 8 and 18, and found that athletes who spend more hours per week playing their sport than their age are 70% more likely to experience a severe injury. In addition, Holt and colleagues[27] found that youth athletes of higher socioeconomic status (and with private health insurance) suffered more serious overuse injuries, particularly because they were the group that demonstrated a trend toward more sports specialization and less free play. Combined with the risks of social isolation, overdependence, burnout, and manipulation,[16,17,28] the benefits of single sport specialization must be carefully considered within the context of the published risk, many of which are discussed in detail herein.

ANATOMY AND PHYSIOLOGY OF THE PEDIATRIC ATHLETE

To more fully understand the potential consequences of single sport specialization on the pediatric and adolescent athlete, it is first critical to understand the physiologic and structural differences between the immature and mature athlete. Although there is no consensus on when sport specialization can safely occur, the age of 12 is generally used as a rough cutoff. This point is largely the age at which puberty and skeletal maturation begins.[28]

From a physiologic standpoint, aerobic (Vo_2 max) and anaerobic capacity increase with age, youth athletes have a higher metabolic cost of running compared with adults, and they have more difficulty dealing with thermoregulation.[29,30] These are critical to understand when treating athletes who may be subjecting themselves to the intense demands of single specialization beyond the more commonly known overuse syndromes discussed herein.

From an orthopedic standpoint, the adolescent growth spurt is a critical time for athletic specialization. During this period, there exists a high risk of injury,[31] particularly involving the apophysis and physis,[32–34] when repetitive activity is performed. Multiple studies have demonstrated that the cartilage present about the physis, apophysis, and articular surfaces are more prone to injury (owing to a decreased resistance to force) during rapid growth phases.[35–37] This is particularly demonstrated by the predisposition of athletes of this age group to suffer injuries to the apophyseal, physeal, and cartilaginous regions (ie, gymnast wrist, Osgood-Schlatter disease, osteochondral lesions).

Hawkins and Metheny[38] outline the following concepts regarding these injuries. It is during rapid periods of growth that muscles and tendons lengthen, yet muscle hypertrophy does not occur at the same rate. As a result, muscles need to produce a greater percentage of their maximal force to produce the same movements that occurred before the growth spurt. This increased force is seen by the tendons. As an example, Hawkins and Metheny[38] calculated that 30% more muscular force is potentially required to develop the same lower leg angular acceleration for an activity such as kicking a ball after a growth spurt as compared with before the growth spurt. If an athlete can generate this force, it is then also transferred to tendons and subsequently the apophyses, potentially leading to overuse injuries if the activity is performed repetitively. If these principles are understood, activities such as strength training can be performed as long as a preparticipation medical evaluation takes place, overall body conditioning is emphasized, and maximal lifts and power lifting are avoided until skeletal maturity is achieved.[39]

The unique anatomy and physiology of the growing athlete places them at a baseline injury risk, which is multiplied by engaging in repetitive, intense activity that can occur with sport specialization.

CONSEQUENCES OF SINGLE SPORT SPECIALIZATION
Physical

Single sport specialization alone is not a problem; rather, the intensive, year-round training in a single sport at the exclusion of other sports causes these issues.[28] Continuous single sport participation subjects the body to the same, repetitive microtrauma and overuse. General guidelines to avoid problems include limiting overall weekly and yearly participation time, limiting repetitive movement (eg, pitching counts), and allowing for scheduled rest periods and/or cross-training during "rest" periods.[28] These recommendations must be individualized based on the athlete, their stage of skeletal maturity (especially during the adolescent growth spurt), and overall conditioning. When uncontrolled or unregulated training occurs, there are serious physical, emotional, and social consequences for both immediate and long-term sports participation.

There is a clear correlation in the literature between training volume and intensity and injury risk, particularly overuse injuries. In fact, the vast majority of injuries seen in a typical sports medicine clinic treating patients from ages 6 to 18 are related to overuse, up to 54.4% in some studies.[40] Furthermore, according to Rose and colleagues[41] in a study of 2721 high school athletes, there was a direct correlation of injury risk with increased weekly hours of sports participation. It therefore follows that, with single sport specialization, there not only exists a greater intensity and volume of training, but also an intensity and volume of training that is repetitive and leads to microtrauma.

For example, Jayanthi and colleagues[11] found that in junior elite tennis players the risk of a reported injury was 1.5 times more likely if they specialized only in tennis. Pitching represents perhaps an even more extraordinary case. Fleisig and colleagues[42] examined 481 youth pitchers (ages 9–14) over a 10-year period and found that pitching more than 100 innings per year increased injury risk 3.5 times. This effect of overuse is further exemplified in a case control study that compared injured and noninjured adolescent pitchers. The study found that the injured group pitched significantly more months per year, games per year, innings per game, pitches per game, pitches per year, and warmup pitches before a game. These pitchers were also more frequently starting pitchers, pitched in more showcases, pitched with higher velocity, and pitched more often with arm pain and fatigue.[43] Clearly, specialization and injury risk are linked.

With regard to the specific injuries seen, the areas of the body that are most prone to overuse injury from repetitive trauma from single sport specialization in the growing athletes, as mentioned previously, are the apophysis and physis.[32–34] This concentration leads to a spectrum of common conditions, including Osgood-Schlatter disease (tibia tubercle apophysitis),[44] Sever disease (calcaneal apophysitis),[45] and Little League elbow (medial epicondyle apophysitis).[46] Physeal injuries such as Little League shoulder (proximal humeral physis)[47] and gymnast wrist (distal radius physis)[48] are also part of this spectrum of injury. Injuries to the cartilage of developing joint surfaces (osteochondral lesion) can also occur. As patients mature, they become more susceptible to adult injury patterns, including stress reactions and stress fractures of the spine (spondylolysis), femoral neck, patella, anterior tibia, medial malleolus, and foot (**Box 1**).[28,49–54]

Two specific areas of concern that have arisen with the increase in single sport specialization and warrant special consideration are the increasing rate of ulnar collateral ligament injuries in pitchers and traumatic knee injuries (ie, anterior cruciate ligament [ACL] tears). An increasing number of ulnar collateral ligament injuries are being seen in patients in younger and younger ages with specialization and overuse cited as the main culprits.[55–59]

From a knee standpoint, Hall and colleagues[60] examined 546 female basketball, soccer, and volleyball players, and found that those athletes involved in a single sport had 1.5-fold relative risk increased risk of patellofemoral pain, Osgood-Schlatter disease, and Sinding Larsen-Johansson syndrome compared with multisport athletes. This distinction is critical, because it has been noted that, among middle and high school female patients with patellofemoral pain, a potential association exists between the development of patellofemoral pain and a subsequent risk of developing ACL injuries later in adolescence.[61] This observation is made in the context of a youth sporting environment that has seen a rapid increase in the incidence of pediatric and adolescent ACL injuries.[62] The increased rate of ACL injury in the young age group has been attributed to early, single sport specialization coupled with a demand for peak performance during a time of change, particularly physiologically, when neuromuscular control and physical fitness may be lacking.[63]

Emotional

Although there is a tendency to concentrate on the physical manifestations of specialization, the psychosocial factors play as important, if not more important, role. Malina[17] described social isolation, overdependence, and burnout as potential consequences (**Box 2**).

Box 1
Common overuse injuries in the single sport athlete

Physical
- Osgood-Schlatter disease
- Sever disease
- Medial epicondyle apophysitis
- Distal radial physeal stress syndrome
- Proximal humeral physiolysis
- Stress fracture (ie, spondylolysis)

Emotional
- Burnout
- Social isolation
- Overdependence

Box 2
Red flags on in-office assessment of the single sport athlete

History
- Decreased performance despite weeks to months of recovery
- Mood disturbances
- Lack of enjoyment in sport
- Presence of triggers such as high training volumes, high time demands, monotony of training, excessive number of competitions.

Physical Examination
- Muscle tightness (positive Ober test, positive Thomas test, popliteal angle >25, ankle dorsiflexion <5, glenohumeral internal rotation deficit)
- Ligamentous laxity
- Q angle greater than 20
- Valgus knee collapse on single leg squat test

From an isolation perspective, the sheer number of hours that youth dedicate to their singular sporting endeavor limits their experiences with other children of their age group who may play other sports and/or no sports at all. In addition, particularly in sports such as gymnastics, home schooling is becoming increasing common, which potentially limits nonathletic interactions with other peers.

From an overdependence perspective, Malina[17] describes the extreme regulation of a young athlete's life in which "overdependence on others" and "loss of control of what is happening in life" can occur. Although not formally studied in a large group of young elite athletes, the constant scheduling of activities by adult influences (ie, parents, coaches, tournament directors) and an overexaggeration of self-worth (ie, "you are special because you excel in a sport") can also potentially negatively affect the young athlete who begins to specialize (and succeed) at a young age.

Burnout is perhaps the most studied consequence of specialization. Burnout has been defined by Smith[64] as a response to chronic stress when a previously enjoyable activity is no longer so. Multiple studies have suggested that early sport specialization can lead to premature cessation of participation either through injury or burnout.[65–67] A recent study by Simon and Docherty[68] looking at former division I collegiate athletes compared with noncollegiate athletes found overall scores lower for athletes on the Patient-Reported Outcomes Measurement Information System for physical function, depression, fatigue, sleep disturbances, and pain interference. This has also been seen by a study performed by Weigand and colleagues,[69] which found higher rates of depression in current college athletes (16.77%) versus former, graduated college athletes (8.03%). In addition, Yang and colleagues[70] found a 21% rate of depression in Division I athletes, particularly among freshman and females.

The sports specialization environment that defines elite performance as success includes high training and time demands, frequent competition, demanding performance expectations, inconsistent coaching practices, little personal control in decision making, negative performance evaluations, the need for perfectionism, the need to please, nonassertiveness, low self-esteem, high anxiety, and an unhealthy focus solely on individual athletic involvement.[17,28,71] A culture has been created in which sports have been transformed from enjoyable to an anxiety-provoking and stressful activity, leading to early departure from sport for many young athletes.

IN-OFFICE ASSESSMENT OF THE SINGLE SPORT PEDIATRIC ATHLETE
Overuse Injuries and Burnout

The in-office assessment of the single sport pediatric athlete should focus on signs of overuse and burnout. Overuse injuries occur owing to repeated submaximal loading of the musculoskeletal system with inadequate rest that prevents structural adaptation and healing. This process damages the muscle–tendon unit, bone, bursa, or neurovascular structures. Approximately 50% of all injuries seen in pediatric sports medicine are related to overuse.[28] Children may be at risk for overuse injuries owing to improper technique, poorly fitting protective equipment, training errors, and muscle weakness and imbalance.[72] There are 4 stages of overuse, in increasing severity: (1) pain in the affected area after physical activity, (2) pain during the activity, without restricting performance, (3) pain during the activity that restricts performance, and (4) chronic, unremitting pain even at rest.[73]

Burnout, also known as overtraining syndrome, failure adaptation, under recovery, or training stress syndrome, is well-described in the adult literature. It is a maladaptive response to excessive exercise that is not matched to appropriate rest, and it represents a systemic inflammatory process with diffuse effects on the neurohormonal axis affecting host immunology and mood. Potential triggers include increased training load without adequate recovery, monotony of training, and excessive number of competitions. The clinical diagnoses is accomplished through history demonstrating (1) decreased performance persisting despite weeks to months of recovery, (2) disturbances in mood, and (3) lack of sign/symptoms or diagnosis of other possible causes of underperformance.[74] Common manifestations in the pediatric athlete include chronic muscle or joint pain, personality changes, elevated resting heart rate, fatigue, lack of enthusiasm about practice or competition, or difficulty with successfully completing usual routines.[73]

When counseling in the clinic, the physician must recognize that there are no scientifically determined guidelines to define how much exercise is healthy and beneficial to the young athlete compared with what might put them at risk for overuse injuries and burnout. The American Academy of Pediatrics Council on Sports Medicine and Fitness recommends limiting one sporting activity to a maximum of 5 days per week with at least 1 day off from any organized activity. Athletes should also have at least 2 to 3 months off per year from their particular sport so that they can let injuries heal, refresh the mind, and work on strength, conditioning, and proprioception in hopes of reducing injury risk.[73] Additionally, youth athletes should have at least 7 hours of sleep each day.[40]

Clinical Examination

In 1992, 5 medical societies—American Academy of Family Physicians, American Academy of Pediatrics, American Medical Society of Sports Medicine, American Orthopedic Society for Sports Medicine, and American Osteopathic Academy of Sports Medicine—collaborated to develop the Preparticipation Physical Examination. Now in its fourth edition, it is widely used to detect potentially life-threatening medical conditions and screen athletes for risk factors that may predispose them to injury or illness.[75] The medical history includes 50 questions and is the most sensitive and specific component of the Preparticipation Physical Examination; it can identify more than 75% of important orthopedic conditions affecting youth athletes.[75]

Beyond the Preparticipation Physical Examination, there are key history questions and physical examination maneuvers to screen for overuse injury and burnout in the single sport youth athlete (see **Box 2**). This includes assessment of athlete happiness and fatigue, parental pressure, and coach involvement, as well as the athlete's training workload, schedule, and equipment. Children or their parents may complain of unexplained underperformance.[74] Questions should include hours per week of activity as well as specifics such as miles per week of running or number of pitches per week. It is important to ask about the number of days off from structured activity, how many different teams the athlete is playing on, any use of supplements, and time spent on strength training, drills, and free play.

The physical examination starts when then patient enters the office with assessment of gait, because an antalgic gait is an immediate marker of injury. Otherwise, depending on the sport, specific areas to focus on for overuse injury are the lateral shoulder, medial elbow, lower back, anterior knee, lower leg, and heel. Point tenderness can be helpful for discerning certain apophyseal and physeal injuries such as Sever disease, Osgood-Schlatter disease, and Little League shoulder.[72,76]

In asymptomatic single sports athletes, there are specific maneuvers to determine those who may be at risk for injury. Boys and girls with a combination of muscle weakness, ligamentous laxity, and muscle tightness are at increased risk for overuse injuries. These overuse effects can be intensified by large body weight and length, high explosive strength, and lower limb malalignment.[77]

The single leg squat test identifies core strength and generally relates to landing, running, and cutting tasks. This maneuver has been shown to correlate well with 2-dimensional, frontal plane video of middle and high school athletes, and is a reasonable tool to assess dynamic knee valgus.[78] Dynamic knee valgus is associated with an increased risk of ACL injury.[79] Hip abduction, extension, and external rotation strength should also be evaluated because there is evidence that hip muscle weakness correlates with conditions such as patellofemoral pain syndrome and iliotibial band syndrome.[80] Additionally, the quadriceps angle can correlate with knee injury. In a prospective cohort study of 400 high school cross-country runners, a quadriceps angle of greater than 20° was associated with a 1.7 times greater risk of injury compared with runners with a quadriceps angle of 10° to 15° ($P<.05$).[81]

In several studies, generalized joint hypermobility has been shown to relate to insidious onset arthralgias, coordination problems, and exercise-related pain.[82,83] Screening for hypermobility has been standardized via the Beighton and Horan Joint Mobility Index, which combines thumb abduction, fifth metacarpal extension, elbow extension, hip flexion, and knee extension for a numerical score.[84]

Muscle tightness has also been shown to relate to injury. A study of 201 collegiate athletes showed that risk of injury increased 23% for each additional point on a 10-point muscle tightness scale (10 = all muscles tight).[85] Lower extremity muscle tightness can be measured in several ways: (1) the Ober test for the iliotibial band, (2) the Thomas test for the iliopsoas, (3) popliteal angle for the hamstring, and (4) ankle dorsiflexion for the gastrocsoleus. In overhead athletes, elbow range of motion and shoulder glenohumeral internal rotation deficit should be checked. Glenohumeral internal rotation deficit is a side-to-side asymmetry of more than 25° produced by acquired posterior capsular contracture or muscle stiffness, and is associated with various shoulder injuries in overhead athletes.[86]

Although history and physical examination are essential in the assessment of the single sport athlete, imaging can play an important role in diagnosis of injury. Imaging for stress reactions, stress fractures, and physeal or apophyseal injuries begins with radiographs, although early radiographs may detect as few as 15% of these injuries in the acute setting.[87] MRI thus offers an advantage over plain radiographs for early detection of these pathologies. MRI can also assist diagnosis of osteochondritis dissecans, ligamentous injury, and tendinopathies. CT has a limited role in diagnosis for overuse injuries, and even in cases of spondylolysis, where CT was previously the gold standard, MRI has been shown to be more sensitive.[88]

ADULT CONSEQUENCES OF SINGLE SPORT SPECIALIZATION

Single sport specialization in the pediatric athlete can have lifelong consequences. For a few examples, we review common pediatric injuries that may occur in the single sport athlete, namely, ulnar collateral ligament tears of the elbow, ACL tears, and spondylolysis.

Ulnar collateral ligament insufficiency is a potentially career-threatening, or even career-ending, injury, particularly for the overhead throwing athlete. In the 1960s, before recognition of the ulnar collateral ligament, professional pitchers were often found to have adaptive changes secondary to prolonged and repetitive throwing, such as flexion contracture, hypertrophy of the dominant extremity, and valgus deformity of the elbow, and nearly 67% of pitchers had radiographic evidence of degenerative elbow disease.[89] If ulnar collateral ligament injuries are managed nonoperatively, only 40% to 50% of high demand throwers can return to play after an average of 6 months away from sport.[90,91] Even with surgery, studies have shown that as many as 26% of high school athletes cannot return to preinjury level of play.[56]

ACL injuries in the pediatric athlete also can have devastating consequences. The association of ACL tears with meniscal injury, and the relation between meniscal loss and degenerative knee arthritis, is well-described in the adult literature.[92] There are fewer pediatric studies, but early data suggest similar associations. In a study by Samora and colleagues[93] of 124 patients, lateral meniscal tears were found in 57% of patients and medial meniscal tears in 29%. There is an increased incidence of medial meniscal injury at the time of ACL surgery when patients are treated for longer than 6 weeks after injury.[92,94] Dumont and colleagues[92] also found that chondral injuries after ACL tear were highly correlated with coexisting meniscal tears, with the medial femoral condyle having the highest rate of injury—over 40% in youth 15 years or older with an ACL tear. These pediatric studies demonstrate the need for early surgery in youth with ACL tears, and show that ACL tears are accompanied by pathology that has potentially long-lasting impact on the life of the knee.

Children generally do well in the short term after conservative management for spondylolysis. A recent meta-analysis demonstrated that 84% of patients managed nonoperatively are able to return to pain-free or near pain-free unrestricted activities. This is despite a lack in radiographic healing, where 71% of unilateral and only 18% of bilateral lesions were found to heal on imaging.[95] Long-term studies show favorable outcomes for patients up to 11 years after diagnosis. However, it is unknown if these patients do well beyond their mid 20s. Patients with spondyloysis on plain radiographs over the age of 25 have more severe disk degeneration below the level of the defect than the general population, which suggests that children with persistent defects on radiographs may eventually have deterioration of function from disk disease.[96]

From just these examples, we see the potential consequences of injury in the pediatric athlete. With the rise of single sport specialization, these injuries are becoming even more common, and thus their effects are even more important. Proper education of athletes, parents, and coaches will allow for the prevention of these injuries.[97] Perhaps the most important concept that all involved should embrace is that a child complaining of pain should seek medical attention. The concept of "pushing through the pain" should not be mandated in youth athletics. With the proper education and utilization of a multidisciplinary team (including parents, coaches, psychologists, and nutritionists) a safe, enjoyable environment for our young athletes can be created.

SUMMARY

Early single sport specialization is an increasing problem among youth athletes and has not been shown to improve long-term athletic performance. There are multiple physical and emotional consequences for engagement in this form of repetitive microtrauma. It is essential for the clinician to understand the differences in adult and youth structure and physiology, particularly during the adolescent growth spurt when injury risk is high. A careful in-office assessment of these athletes with an understanding of the potential long-term consequences of early specialization is critical.

REFERENCES

1. National Council on Youth Sports. Report on trends and participation in organized youth sports. 2008. Available at: http://www.ncys.org/pdfs/2008/2008-ncys-market-research-report.pdf.
2. Kann L, Kinchen S, Shanklin SL, et al. Youth risk behavior surveillance–United States, 2013. MMWR Surveill Summ 2014;63(Suppl 4):1–168.

3. Kelley B, Carchia C. "Hey, data data – swing!". ESPN The Magazine 2013.

4. Epstein D. Hyperspecialization is ruining youth sports—and the kids who play them. 2014. Available at: http://www.propublica.org/article/hyperspecialization-is-ruining-youth-sportsand-the-kids-who-play-them. Accessed October 16, 2014.

5. Hyman M. The most expensive game in town. The rising cost of youth sports and the toll on today's families. Boston: Beacon Press; 2012.

6. Lykissas MG, Eismann EA, Parikh SN. Trends in pediatric sports-related and recreation-related Injuries in the United States in the last decade. J Pediatr Orthop 2013;33:803–10.

7. Ericsson K, Krampe R, Tesch-Romer C. The role of deliberate practice in the acquisition of expert performance. Psychol Rev 1993;100:363–406.

8. Hill G, Simons J. A study of the sport specialization on high school athletics. J Sport Social Iss 1989;13:1–13.

9. Metzl JD. Expectations of pediatric sport participation among pediatricians, patients, and parents. Pediatr Clin North Am 2002;49:497–504, v.

10. Wiersma L. Risks and benefits of youth sport specialization: perspectives and recommendations. Pediatr Exerc Sci 2000;12:13–22.

11. Jayanthi N, Dechert A, Durazo R, et al. Training and specialization risks in junior elite tennis players. J Med Sci Tennis 2011;16:14–20.

12. American College of Sports Medicine. Current comment from the American College of Sports Medicine. August 1993–"The prevention of sport injuries of children and adolescents". Med Sci Sports Exerc 1993;25:1–7.

13. DiFiori J. Overuse injuries in young athletes: an overview. Athl Ther Today 2002;7:25.

14. Micheli LJ, Glassman R, Klein M. The prevention of sports injuries in children. Clin Sports Med 2000; 19:821–34, ix.

15. American Academy of Pediatrics. Intensive training and sports specialization in young athletes. American Academy of Pediatrics. Committee on Sports Medicine and Fitness. Pediatrics 2000;106:154–7.

16. Jayanthi N, Pinkham C, Dugas L, et al. Sports specialization in young athletes: evidence-based recommendations. Sports Health 2013;5:251–7.

17. Malina RM. Early sport specialization: roots, effectiveness, risks. Curr Sports Med Rep 2010;9:364–71.

18. Probability of competing beyond high school. 2013. Available at: http://www.ncaa.org/about/resources/research/probability-competing-beyond-high-school. Accessed October 16, 2014.

19. Pennington B. The scholarship divide. Expectations lose to reality of sports scholarships. 2008. Available at: http://www.nytimes.com/2008/03/10/sports/10scholarships.html?_r=2&adxnnl=1&oref=,&adxnnlx=1413459840-OTiOGVzEKvyYuiCV5wXHLg. Accessed October 16, 2014.

20. Abernathy B, Baker J, Cote. Transfer of pattern recall skills may contribute to the development of sport expertise. Appl Cognit Psychol 2005;19:705–18.

21. Fransen J, Pion J, Vandendriessche J, et al. Differences in physical fitness and gross motor coordination in boys aged 6-12 years specializing in one versus sampling more than one sport. J Sports Sci 2012;30:379–86.

22. Gullich A, Emrich E. Evaluation of the support of young athletes in the elite sports system. Eur J Sport Soc 2006;3:85–108.

23. Gullich A, Emrich E. Individualistic and collectivistic approach in athlete support programmes in the German high-performance sport system. Eur J Sport Soc 2012;9:243–68.

24. DiFiori J. Early sports participation: a prescription for success? Presented at the 2013 American Medical Society for Sports Medicine National Meeting. San Diego, April 17–21, 2013.

25. Vaeyens R, Gullich A, Warr CR, et al. Talent identification and promotion programmes of Olympic athletes. J Sports Sci 2009;27:1367–80.

26. Jayanthi N, LaBella C, Dugas L, et al. Risks of specialized training and growth for injury in young athletes: a prospective cohort study. Presented at the American Academy of Pediatrics National Meeting. Orlando, October 24–27, 2013.

27. Holt D, Jayanthi N, Austin A, et al. Socioeconomic factors for sports specialization and injury in young athletes: a clinical study. Presented at the American Academy of Pediatrics National Meeting. San Diego, October 11–14, 2014.

28. DiFiori JP, Benjamin HJ, Brenner JS, et al. Overuse injuries and burnout in youth sports: a position statement from the American Medical Society for Sports Medicine. Br J Sports Med 2014;48:287–8.

29. Bar-Or O. The young athlete: some physiological considerations. J Sports Sci 1995;13(Spec No): S31–3.

30. Zauner CW, Maksud MG, Melichna J. Physiological considerations in training young athletes. Sports Med 1989;8:15–31.

31. Caine D, Cochrane B, Caine C, et al. An epidemiologic investigation of injuries affecting young competitive female gymnasts. Am J Sports Med 1989;17:811–20.

32. Caine D, DiFiori J, Maffulli N. Physeal injuries in children's and youth sports: reasons for concern? Br J Sports Med 2006;40:749–60.

33. Difiori JP. Overuse injury of the physis: a "growing" problem. Clin J Sport Med 2010;20:336–7.

34. DiFiori JP. Evaluation of overuse injuries in children and adolescents. Curr Sports Med Rep 2010;9: 372–8.

35. Alexander C. Effects of growth rate on the strength of the growth plate-shaft junction. Skeletal Radiol 1976;1:67–76.

36. Bright RW, Burstein AH, Elmore SM. Epiphyseal-plate cartilage. A biomechanical and histological analysis of failure modes. J Bone Joint Surg Am 1974;56:688–703.

37. Flachsmann R, Broom ND, Hardy AE, et al. Why is the adolescent joint particularly susceptible to osteochondral shear fracture? Clin Orthop Relat Res 2000;381:212–21.

38. Hawkins D, Metheny J. Overuse injuries in youth sports: biomechanical considerations. Med Sci Sports Exerc 2001;33:1701–7.

39. Bernhardt DT, Gomez J, Johnson MD, et al. Strength training by children and adolescents. Pediatrics 2001;107:1470–2.

40. Luke A, Lazaro RM, Bergeron MF, et al. Sports-related injuries in youth athletes: is overscheduling a risk factor? Clin J Sport Med 2011;21:307–14.

41. Rose MS, Emery CA, Meeuwisse WH. Sociodemographic predictors of sport injury in adolescents. Med Sci Sports Exerc 2008;40:444–50.

42. Fleisig GS, Andrews JR, Cutter GR, et al. Risk of serious injury for young baseball pitchers: a 10-year prospective study. Am J Sports Med 2011;39:253–7.

43. Olsen SJ 2nd, Fleisig GS, Dun S, et al. Risk factors for shoulder and elbow injuries in adolescent baseball pitchers. Am J Sports Med 2006;34:905–12.

44. Osgood RB. Lesions of the tibial tubercle occurring during adolescence. 1903. Clin Orthop Relat Res 1993;(286):4–9.

45. Sever JW. Apophysitis of the os calcis. New York Medical J 1912;95:1025–9.

46. Benjamin HJ, Briner WW Jr. Little league elbow. Clin J Sport Med 2005;15:37–40.

47. Adams JE. Little league shoulder: osteochondrosis of the proximal humeral epiphysis in boy baseball pitchers. Calif Med 1966;105:22–5.

48. Dobyns JH, Gabel GT. Gymnast's wrist. Hand Clin 1990;6:493–505.

49. Micheli LJ, Wood R. Back pain in young athletes. Significant differences from adults in causes and patterns. Arch Pediatr Adolesc Med 1995;149:15–8.

50. Maezawa K, Nozawa M, Sugimoto M, et al. Stress fractures of the femoral neck in child with open capital femoral epiphysis. J Pediatr Orthop B 2004;13:407–11.

51. Garcia Mata S, Hidalgo Ovejero A, Martinez Grande M. Transverse stress fracture of the patella in a child. J Pediatr Orthop B 1999;8:208–11.

52. Shabat S, Sampson KB, Mann G, et al. Stress fractures of the medial malleolus–review of the literature and report of a 15-year-old elite gymnast. Foot Ankle Int 2002;23:647–50.

53. Beals RK, Cook RD. Stress fractures of the anterior tibial diaphysis. Orthopedics 1991;14:869–75.

54. Ribbans WJ, Natarajan R, Alavala S. Pediatric foot fractures. Clin Orthop Relat Res 2005;432:107–15.

55. American Sports Medicine Institute. Position statement for youth baseball pitchers. 2013. Available at: http://www.asmi.org/research.php?page=research&section=positionStatement. Accessed October 17, 2014.

56. Petty DH, Andrews JR, Fleisig GS, et al. Ulnar collateral ligament reconstruction in high school baseball players: clinical results and injury risk factors. Am J Sports Med 2004;32:1158–64.

57. Savoie FH 3rd, Trenhaile SW, Roberts J, et al. Primary repair of ulnar collateral ligament injuries of the elbow in young athletes: a case series of injuries to the proximal and distal ends of the ligament. Am J Sports Med 2008;36:1066–72.

58. Zell M, Dwek JR, Edmonds EW. Origin of the medial ulnar collateral ligament on the pediatric elbow. J Child Orthop 2013;7:323–8.

59. Larsen N, Moisan A, Witte D, et al. Medial ulnar collateral ligament origin in children and adolescents: an MRI anatomic study. J Pediatr Orthop 2013;33:664–6.

60. Hall R, Barber Foss K, Hewett TE, et al. Sports specialization is associated with an increased risk of developing anterior knee pain in adolescent female athletes. J Sport Rehabil 2014. [Epub ahead of print].

61. Myer GD, Ford KR, Di Stasi SL, et al. High knee abduction moments are common risk factors for patellofemoral pain (PFP) and anterior cruciate ligament (ACL) injury in girls: is PFP itself a predictor for subsequent ACL injury? Br J Sports Med 2014. [Epub ahead of print].

62. Sampson NR, Beck NA, Baldwin KD, et al. Knee injuries in children and adolescents: has there been an increase in ACL and meniscus tears in recent years? Presented at the American Academy of Pediatrics National Meeting. Boston, October 14–18, 2011.

63. Ladenhauf HN, Graziano J, Marx RG. Anterior cruciate ligament prevention strategies: are they effective in young athletes - current concepts and review of literature. Curr Opin Pediatr 2013;25:64–71.

64. Smith R. Toward a cognitive-affective model of athletic burnout. J Sport Psychol 1986;8:36–50.

65. Budgett R. Fatigue and underperformance in athletes: the overtraining syndrome. Br J Sports Med 1998;32:107–10.

66. Wall MC. Developmental activities that lead to dropout and investment in sport. Phys Educ Sport Pedagogy 2007;12:77–87.

67. Gould D, Udry E, Tuffey S, et al. Burnout in competitive junior tennis players: pt. 1. a quantitative psychological assessment. Sport Psychol 1996;10:322–40.

68. Simon JE, Docherty CL. Current health-related quality of life is lower in former Division I collegiate athletes than in non-collegiate athletes. Am J Sports Med 2014;42:423–9.

69. Weigand S, Cohen J, Merenstein D. Susceptibility for depression in current and retired student athletes. Sports Health 2013;5:263–6.

70. Yang J, Peek-Asa C, Corlette JD, et al. Prevalence of and risk factors associated with symptoms of depression in competitive collegiate student athletes. Clin J Sport Med 2007;17:481–7.

71. Matos NF, Winsley RJ, Williams CA. Prevalence of nonfunctional overreaching/overtraining in young English athletes. Med Sci Sports Exerc 2011;43:1287–94.

72. Cassas KJ, Cassettari-Wayhs A. Childhood and adolescent sports-related overuse injuries. Am Fam Physician 2006;73:1014–22.

73. Brenner JS, American Academy of Pediatrics Council on Sports Medicine and Fitness. Overuse injuries, overtraining, and burnout in child and adolescent athletes. Pediatrics 2007;119:1242–5.

74. Kreher JB, Schwartz JB. Overtraining syndrome: a practical guide. Sports Health 2012;4:128–38.

75. Seto CK. The preparticipation physical examination: an update. Clin Sports Med 2011;30:491–501.

76. Osbahr DC, Kim HJ, Dugas JR. Little league shoulder. Curr Opin Pediatr 2010;22:35–40.

77. Lysens RJ, Ostyn MS, Vanden Auweele Y, et al. The accident-prone and overuse-prone profiles of the young athlete. Am J Sports Med 1989;17:612–9.

78. Ugalde V, Brockman C, Bailowitz Z, et al. Single limb squat test and its relationship to dynamic knee valgus and injury risk screening. PM R 2014. [Epub ahead of print].

79. Hewett TE, Myer GD, Ford KR, et al. Biomechanical measures of neuromuscular control and valgus loading of the knee predict anterior cruciate ligament injury risk in female athletes: a prospective study. Am J Sports Med 2005;33:492–501.

80. Paterno MV, Taylor-Haas JA, Myer GD, et al. Prevention of overuse sports injuries in the young athlete. Orthop Clin North Am 2013;44:553–64.

81. Rauh MJ, Koepsell TD, Rivara FP, et al. Quadriceps angle and risk of injury among high school cross-country runners. J Orthop Sports Phys Ther 2007;37:725–33.

82. Adib N, Davies K, Grahame R, et al. Joint hypermobility syndrome in childhood. A not so benign multisystem disorder? Rheumatology 2005;44:744–50.

83. Valovich McLeod TC, Decoster LC, Loud KJ, et al. National Athletic Trainers' Association position statement: prevention of pediatric overuse injuries. J Athl Train 2011;46:206–20.

84. Beighton P, Horan F. Orthopaedic aspects of the Ehlers-Danlos syndrome. J Bone Joint Surg Br 1969;51:444–53.

85. Krivickas LS, Feinberg JH. Lower extremity injuries in college athletes: relation between ligamentous laxity and lower extremity muscle tightness. Arch Phys Med Rehabil 1996;77:1139–43.

86. Sciascia A, Kibler WB. The pediatric overhead athlete: what is the real problem? Clin J Sport Med 2006;16:471–7.

87. Rauck RC, LaMont LE, Doyle SM. Pediatric upper extremity stress injuries. Curr Opin Pediatr 2013;25:40–5.

88. Rush JK, Astur N, Scott S, et al. The use of magnetic resonance imaging in the evaluation of spondylolysis. J Pediatr Orthop 2014. [Epub ahead of print].

89. Langer P, Fadale P, Hulstyn M. Evolution of the treatment options of ulnar collateral ligament injuries of the elbow. Br J Sports Med 2006;40:499–506.

90. Barnes DA, Tullos HS. An analysis of 100 symptomatic baseball players. Am J Sports Med 1978;6:62–7.

91. Rettig AC, Sherrill C, Snead DS, et al. Nonoperative treatment of ulnar collateral ligament injuries in throwing athletes. Am J Sports Med 2001;29:15–7.

92. Dumont GD, Hogue GD, Padalecki JR, et al. Meniscal and chondral injuries associated with pediatric anterior cruciate ligament tears: relationship of treatment time and patient-specific factors. Am J Sports Med 2012;40:2128–33.

93. Samora WP 3rd, Palmer R, Klingele KE. Meniscal pathology associated with acute anterior cruciate ligament tears in patients with open physes. J Pediatr Orthop 2011;31:272–6.

94. Millett PJ, Willis AA, Warren RF. Associated injuries in pediatric and adolescent anterior cruciate ligament tears: does a delay in treatment increase the risk of meniscal tear? Arthroscopy 2002;18:955–9.

95. Klein G, Mehlman CT, McCarty M. Nonoperative treatment of spondylolysis and grade I spondylolisthesis in children and young adults: a meta-analysis of observational studies. J Pediatr Orthop 2009;29:146–56.

96. Miller SF, Congeni J, Swanson K. Long-term functional and anatomical follow-up of early detected spondylolysis in young athletes. Am J Sports Med 2004;32:928–33.

97. Stop Sports Injuries. Available at: http://www.stopsportsinjuries.org/sports-injury-prevention.aspx. Accessed October 27, 2014.

Upper Extremity

Preface
Upper Extremity

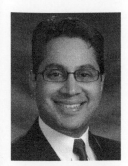

Asif M. Ilyas, MD
Editor

In this issue of the *Orthopedic Clinics of North America*, we present several interesting articles in the Upper Extremity section reviewing a broad range of topics.

Distal radius fractures are among the most common fractures seen and managed in the emergency department. However, some controversy still exists on its acute management. Padegimas and Ilyas present a practical review of emergency department management of distal radius fractures, including physical examination, radiographic diagnosis, closed reduction and splinting techniques, as well as surgical indications.

Elbow instability encompasses a wide variety of traumatic conditions of the elbow ranging from simple acute dislocations to complex ones with a combination of bony and ligamentous injuries. These are challenging injuries where treatment is predicated on both accurate diagnosis and timely treatment. Ahmed and Mistry present a detailed review, including diagnosis and the full spectrum of treatment options for both acute and chronic cases.

Thumb ulnar collateral ligament injuries are common conditions that can be a product of chronic trauma, but more commonly, acute trauma. Avery and colleagues provide a detailed review of this condition, including physical examination, diagnosis, and management.

Rotator cuff calcific tendinopathy is a relatively uncommon but interesting condition that is often found incidentally on radiographs during evaluation of shoulder pain. Greis and colleagues provide a comprehensive review of this tendinopathy, including its pathophysiology, diagnosis, and nonoperative management, including ultrasound-guided lavage and extracorporeal shock-wave therapy.

Asif M. Ilyas, MD
Hand & Upper Extremity Surgery
Rothman Institute
Thomas Jefferson University
925 Chestnut Street
Philadelphia, PA 19107, USA

E-mail address:
asif.ilyas@rothmaninstitute.com

Orthop Clin N Am 46 (2015) xxi
http://dx.doi.org/10.1016/j.ocl.2014.12.001
0030-5898/15/$ – see front matter © 2015 Published by Elsevier Inc.

Distal Radius Fractures
Emergency Department Evaluation and Management

Eric M. Padegimas, MD*, Asif M. Ilyas, MD

KEYWORDS

- Distal radius fracture • Emergency department • Hematoma block • Splinting

KEY POINTS

- Diagnosis of a distal radius fracture can be made readily with plain radiographs and does not routinely require advanced imaging with computed tomography or MRI.
- Findings that may warrant urgent surgical management include an open fracture, vascular injury, or acute carpal tunnel syndrome.
- Indications for emergency department reduction include significant deformity, joint dislocation or subluxation, and radiographic parameters that include more than 20 degrees of dorsal tilt.
- On reduction, casting should be avoided and ace compression wrapping over the splint should be applied loosely allowing for early and free finger motion.
- Outpatient surgical indications are based on a variety of factors including patient demographics, age, concomitant injuries, fracture alignment, and fracture stability.

INTRODUCTION

Musculoskeletal injuries, such as distal radius fractures of the wrist, are a common presentation to an emergency department (ED). In the United States, these injuries are second only to respiratory illnesses in frequency of ED visits, accounting for 20% of chief complaints.[1–3] However, despite the frequency of presentation, education in musculoskeletal injuries is often considered deficient in medical education.[4–8] The volume of orthopedic presentations to an ED prompted further study of musculoskeletal education in emergency medicine training.[3] Comer and colleagues[3] provided a validated 25-question orthopedic examination published in 1998 by Freedman and Bernstein to emergency medicine residents and attendings at all levels of training. The results found a 61% overall passing rate (65% for residents and 57% for attendings). As a result of the frequency of musculoskeletal injuries, it is important for all practitioners who evaluate or treat patients in the ED to be well-educated in these injuries.

Distal radius fractures are the most common upper extremity fracture affecting all patient populations, but are particularly prevalent in the young and elderly.[9] Among patients older than 65 years of age, distal radius fractures account for 18% of all fractures.[10] This injury is seen by orthopedic surgeons with an incidence of 195.2 per 100,000 patients per year.[11] The active elderly are disproportionately affected because the common mechanism of the fracture is a standing level fall onto an outstretched hand. The health burden of this injury pattern is substantial because there were 640,000 reported distal radius fractures in the United States in 2001.[12,13] There is also a significant economic burden because distal radius fractures contribute significantly to the approximate $1.1 billion cost of osteoporotic fractures in the Medicare population.[14,15] Furthermore, the incidence of this injury pattern has been on the rise in the United States and internationally, with a

Department of Orthopaedic Surgery, Thomas Jefferson University Hospital, 111 South 11th St, Philadelphia, PA 19107, USA
* Corresponding author.
E-mail address: padegimase@gmail.com

Orthop Clin N Am 46 (2015) 259–270
http://dx.doi.org/10.1016/j.ocl.2014.11.010
0030-5898/15/$ – see front matter © 2015 Elsevier Inc. All rights reserved.

orthopedic.theclinics.com

disproportionate increase in patients 65 years and older.[13,16–20] As life expectancy continues to rise and people remain active later in life, distal radius fractures will be an increasingly significant clinical problem.[21,22]

This article provides an evidence-based guide of early management of distal radius fractures. This is intended for practitioners who would treat this injury in an ED. We discuss the typical presentation of distal radius fractures, radiographic findings, and early management strategies, and focus on what emergent situations require immediate orthopedic intervention.

HISTORY AND PHYSICAL EXAMINATION

When assessing the patient who sustains a wrist injury, history and physical examination are an important diagnostic tool. The classic presentation of distal radius fractures is the elderly female with a fall onto an outstretched hand.[23–30] However, unlike these relatively low-energy injuries that typically occur from falling from a standing level, higher-energy injuries can also result in distal radius fractures with a higher prevalence in younger populations. A full trauma assessment of these patients is often necessary because the wrist fracture may not be an isolated injury.

The first step in physical examination is assessment for any obvious deformity. Most displaced fractures present with a wrist that is swollen and potentially deformed and angulated (**Fig. 1**). Concurrently, the skin and soft tissue should be examined for any defects that could generate concern for an open fracture (**Fig. 2**). Patients

with an open fracture should also be treated with tetanus prophylaxis (based on patient's immunization status) and intravenous antibiotics immediately.[31–33]

Vascular examination is the next component of the examination. The hand and wrist is well perfused with robust vascular anatomy. Capillary refill of the finger tips is a common technique used to evaluate blood flow of the hand but has low sensitivity in confirming perfusion. Moreover, it is commonly delayed because of swelling and deformity, but radial and ulnar pulses should be palpable. If pulses are not palpable, the deformity can be improved and the vascular examination can be repeated. Alternatively, consider using a Doppler ultrasound. If pulses are still not present and/or if there is concern for a vascular injury, such as ischemic changes to the hand, rapidly enlarging hematoma, or the presence of arterial bleeding, consider emergent evaluation by an orthopedic surgeon or a vascular surgeon.

Neurologic examination is often difficult to assess in the setting of an acute fracture because of pain. Moreover, patient discrimination between subjective pain, numbness, and paresthesia may be highly variable. Nonetheless, a thorough examination of the hand with careful assessment of sensory and motor function of the radial, median, and ulnar nerves is critical. The radial nerve can be tested for sensation on the dorsal aspect of the first webspace of the hand, whereas motor function is assessed by thumb and finger extension testing. Sensation in the ulnar nerve can be tested on the palmar aspect of the small finger and motor innervation is tested by assessing finger

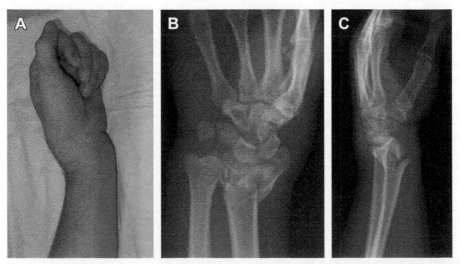

Fig. 1. (A) Typical deformity of a distal radius fracture with dorsal angulation and swelling. Note the associated distal radius fracture on (B) posteroanterior and (C) lateral views.

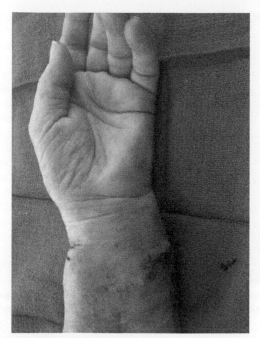

Fig. 2. Soft tissue defects about the wrist should arouse concern for an open fracture.

abduction. Sensation in the median nerve can be tested on the palmar aspect of the index finger (**Fig. 3**A) and motor innervation is tested by assessing thumb abduction, specifically the abductor pollicis brevis (see **Fig. 3**B).[34] Although neurologic examination may be limited secondary to pain and swelling, the median nerve is at particular risk of injury with a displaced distal radius fracture and its dysfunction must be readily recognized (**Fig. 4**). Median nerve dysfunction

may be a result of nerve contusion or acute carpal tunnel syndrome.[35] Median nerve contusion is a nonemergent condition consisting of nonprogressive numbness in the sensory distribution of the median nerve. Conversely, patients with an acute carpal tunnel syndrome present with a rapidly progressive median neuropathy with worsening painful parasthesias in its sensory distribution. This acute compressive neuropathy results from immediate postinjury swelling in the carpal tunnel and is an emergent situation that requires immediate surgical decompression of the median nerve in the carpal tunnel and fracture reduction.[36–41]

RADIOGRAPHIC ANALYSIS

Plain radiographs are the mainstay of diagnosis of distal radius fractures. Standard posteroanterior, lateral, and oblique radiographs are typically sufficient (see **Fig. 1**). There are several radiographic parameters that are important to analyze in distal radius fractures. Variations from these normal parameters may confirm the presence of a fracture. Furthermore, the extent of variation from these parameters can dictate surgical or nonsurgical management of distal radius fractures. These parameters are radial inclination, radial length, volar tilt, ulnar variance, and the scapholunate angle (**Fig. 5**). The normal values for these measurements are approximately 23 degrees for radial inclination, 12 mm for radial length, 10 degrees for volar tilt, and −0.6 mm for ulnar variance.[42,43] Common concomitant injuries to the wrist should also be considered when evaluating radiographs for a possible distal radius fracture, and include other carpal fractures, such as of the scaphoid,

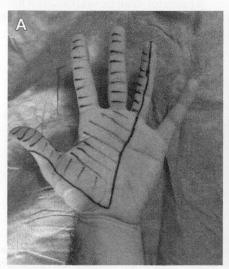
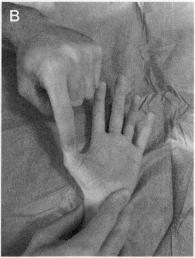

Fig. 3. The median nerve is tested by sensory and motor examination. (*A*) Sensory distribution of the median nerve in the hand is noted by the shaded area. (*B*) Motor examination is best performed by testing thumb abduction stress testing.

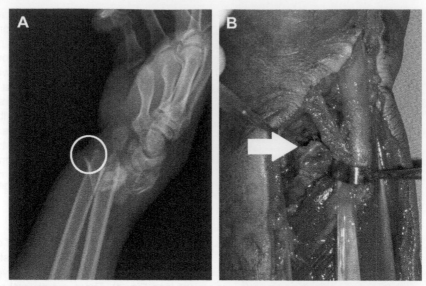

Fig. 4. The risk for median nerve injury is increased with excessive fracture displacement. (*A*) Note the volar spike of the radius on the lateral view (*circle*), and (*B*) the intraoperative finding of direct median nerve compression (*arrow*).

distal ulna fractures, disruption of the distal radio-ulnar and radiocarpal joints, and intercarpal ligament injuries, such as a scapholunate ligament tears or perilunate dislocations (**Fig. 6**).

Advanced imaging is typically not indicated in the acute setting. However, computed tomography scan may be used for preoperative planning of comminuted fractures with articular involvement.[44,45] MRI can be useful to assess for additional internal derangement of the wrist, such as a suspected concomitant ligamentous injury.

OPEN FRACTURE MANAGEMENT

An open fracture of the distal radius should be initially managed as any other open fracture in the ED setting. The patient should be provided with tetanus prophylaxis, receiving either a tetanus toxoid booster or a combination of the booster with human tetanus immunoglobulin, depending on the patient's tetanus prophylaxis history.[46]

Early administration of antibiotics is critical because open fractures are by definition contaminated. Appropriate antibiotics should ideally be administered within 3 hours of the injury to lower infection rate.[33,47] Specific antibiotic therapy depends on the extent of soft tissue injury, which is commonly classified with the Gustilo-Anderson system. Gustilo I fractures require cefazolin every 8 hours for three doses, Gustilo II fractures require cefazolin and tobramycin or piperacillin/tazobactam for 24 hours after wound closure, and Gustilo

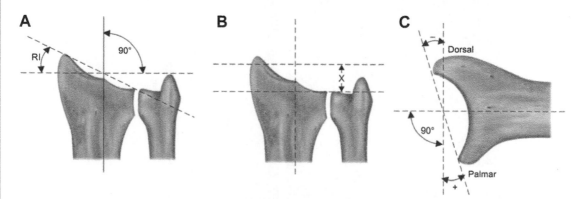

Fig. 5. Standard radiographic measurements of the distal radius include (*A*) radial inclination of approximately 23 degrees, (*B*) radial height of approximately 11 mm, and (*C*) volar tilt of approximately 10 degrees. (*From* Bruinsma W, Peters F, Jupiter J. Distal radius fractures. In: Ilyas A, Rehman S, editors. Contemporary surgical management of fractures and complications. New Delhi (India): Jaypee Brothers Medical Publishers (P) Ltd; 2013. p. 132; with permission.)

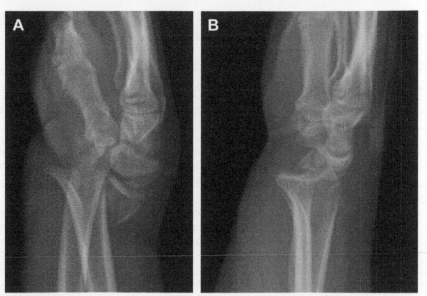

Fig. 6. Differentiating between (*A*) dorsally displaced distal radius fracture and (*B*) dorsally dislocated radiocarpal fracture-dislocation may be difficult. Note the maintenance of most of the native articular surface with the radio-carpal fracture-dislocation, whereas in the case of the distal radius fracture the articular surface displaces with the carpus. (*From* Bruinsma W, Peters F, Jupiter J. Distal radius fractures. In: Ilyas A, Rehman S, editors. Contemporary surgical management of fractures and complications. New Delhi (India): Jaypee Brothers Medical Publishers (P) Ltd; 2013. p. 135; with permission.)

III fractures require cefazolin and tobramycin or piperacillin/tazobactam with the addition of intravenous penicillin if the wound is contaminated with soil (anaerobic coverage) for a minimum of 3 days after wound closure (**Table 1**).[32,48]

An orthopedic surgeon should be consulted immediately for these injuries because these must be treated urgently with operative wound irrigation and debridement. Historically, the goal has been 6 hours to initial debridement[32]; however, strict adherence to the 6-hour goal does not seem to be justified by more recent analysis.[49] Although early intervention is important, emergent debridement and exploration is more frequently reserved for highly contaminated injuries or concomitant vascular injuries that require emergent management. Specifically for open distal radius fractures, the risk of deep infection and fracture nonunion are predicted by Gustilo-Anderson classification rather than time to operating room.[50] In general, the specific operative intervention in open distal radius fractures is determined by the degree of soft tissue damage.[51]

Emergency Department Management

Initial ED management consists of the physical examination including evaluation of the neurovascular status and assessment for open wounds, and radiographic evaluation. Once satisfied with the diagnosis a fracture reduction may be performed.

Indications for Fracture Reduction

An ED reduction of a distal radius fracture is not always necessary. Unless the reduction to be attempted in the ED is the definitive treatment, fractures with minimal deformity, radiographic parameters that include less than 20 degrees of dorsal tilt, minimal displacement, and no joint subluxation or dislocation do not require additional treatment beyond splinting the patient in situ without manipulation. Alternatively, if obvious deformity to the wrist is evident, correction of the deformity is indicated to prevent excessive swelling, late neurovascular compromise, and skin tenting with possible late skin necrosis and wound formation.

Hematoma Block

If a reduction is indicated, it is important for the practitioner to provide adequate analgesia. This is critical for patient comfort and to facilitate fracture reduction. The two most commonly used techniques for analgesia in the ED are sedation or local anesthesia, in the form of a hematoma block. A recent double-blind, randomized clinical trial found conscious sedation to take longer than hematoma block without a significant difference in analgesia or loss of reduction after 1 week.[52]

Table 1
Gustilo-Anderson classification of open fractures and antibiotic recommendations

Classification	Criteria	Description	Antibiotics[a]

Gustilo I	Wound <1 cm
	No contamination
	Simple fracture
	No periosteal stripping
		Local skin coverage
		No neurovascular injury
		Low energy
		No soft tissue damage
			First-generation
			  cephalosporin for 24 h
			  after closure

Gustilo II	Wound >1 cm
	Moderate contamination
	Moderate comminution
	No periosteal stripping
		Local skin coverage
		No neurovascular injury
		Moderate energy
		No extensive soft tissue damage
			First-generation
			  cephalosporin for 24 h
			  after closure

Gustilo III			

IIIA	Large injury zone
	Extensive contamination
	Severe comminution or
	  segmental fracture
	Periosteal stripping
		Local skin coverage
		No neurovascular injury
		High energy
		Extensive soft tissue damage
			First-generation
			  cephalosporin and
			  aminoglycoside (gram-
			  negative) for 24–72 h
			  after debridement

IIIB	Large injury zone
	Extensive contamination
	Severe comminution or
	  segmental fracture
	Periosteal stripping
		Requires soft tissue
		  coverage (flap)
		No neurovascular injury
		High energy
		Extensive soft tissue damage
			First-generation
			  cephalosporin and
			  aminoglycoside (gram-
			  negative) for 24–72 h
			  after debridement

IIIC	Large injury zone
	Extensive contamination
	Severe comminution or
	  segmental fracture
	Periosteal stripping
		Local skin coverage
		Neurovascular injury
		  requiring arterial repair
		High energy
		Extensive soft tissue damage
			First-generation
			  cephalosporin and
			  aminoglycoside (gram-
			  negative) for 24–72 h
			  after debridement

[a] Add high-dose penicillin if agricultural injury with anaerobic concern.

The techniques of conscious sedation are beyond the scope of this article. We instead discuss the technique of a hematoma block because this is a versatile clinical tool and can be performed independently.

A hematoma block is a reliable anesthetic technique that has been well-described in ED fracture management.[53–55] A good neurologic examination should be documented before proceeding because introduction of a local anesthetic may transiently blunt median nerve function and subsequent examination. A hematoma block begins with examining the wrist and radiographs to identify the area of deformity and the subsequent fracture site. Using a 22-gauge needle with 5 to 10 mL of 1% or 2% lidocaine, the needle is directed through the dorsal side of the wrist into the fracture site (**Fig. 7**). Before injecting, hematoma blood aspirate should be drawn back into the syringe to confirm localization of the needle within the fracture hematoma. Once the patient has achieved adequate pain relief, the practitioner may attempt reduction and immobilization. This technique should be used with caution in pediatric patients in fractures with open growth plates because the anesthetic may have a toxic effect on the physis.

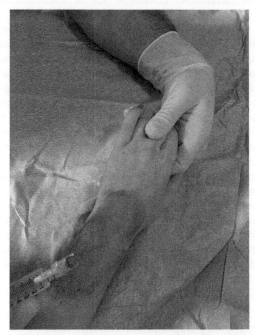

Fig. 7. Hematoma block, injected dorsally after cleaning skin with Betadine or chlorhexidine preparation. Only inject after confirming placement in fracture hematoma with return of a blood aspirate into the syringe.

Fracture Reduction and Splinting

The general principles of distal radius fracture closed reduction are (1) to accentuate the deformity to disengage the fracture fragments, (2) distraction of the fracture site, and (3) correction of the deformity. Specific reduction technique depends on the fracture pattern itself and the direction of the angulation or displacement. Most distal radius fractures are dorsally angulated. Traction can be safely applied manually or with the use of finger traps.[56,57] When using finger traps, reduction can be performed with the patient's arm hanging from the traps and with an assistant pulling countertraction on the arm, or alternatively with weights applied proximally over the arm to provide countertraction independently. Without finger traps, the practitioner should grip the patient's hand as if performing a handshake, extend the wrist to disengage the fracture site, apply axial traction, and then apply a force that is directed volarly and ulnarly while in pronation on the distal fragment (**Fig. 8**).[35] Overflexion should be avoided especially if the radiograph shows a large volar spike (see **Fig. 4**) because excessive flexion can increase the risk of development of acute carpal tunnel syndrome.

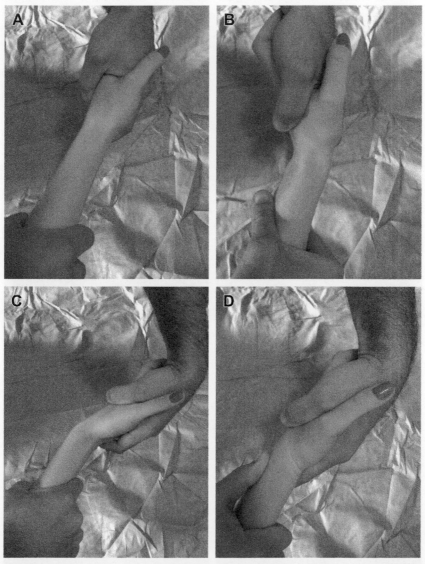

Fig. 8. Reduction maneuver for a typical dorsally angulated distal radius fractures. (*A*) Hold patient's hand as if performing a handshake. (*B*) Axial traction and wrist extension to disengage fracture site. (*C*) Flex the wrist while maintaining axial traction. (*D*) Apply a volarly and ulnarly directed force while in mild pronation.

After performing the reduction maneuver, the fracture must be immobilized. This can be safely done in a sugar-tong splint (**Fig. 9**), a short arm radial gutter splint (**Fig. 10**), or a volar splint (**Fig. 11**).[58] In the acute setting, splinting is preferable to casting because casts may increase risk of pain and complications from swelling in a closed area.[59] After splinting and application of additional Webril over the plaster, ace compression wrapping should be loosely applied. No more than one ace wrap should be applied for a wrist-based splint, and possibly two for a sugar-tong splint. The ace wrap should be applied loosely, from distal to proximal, and overlap no more than 50%. The ace wrap should also include the base of the hand but exclude the fingers. Finger range of motion should be encouraged to improve swelling and avoid stiffness. Excessive or too tight ace wrap application can result in significant pain, swelling, and stiffness postreduction and is among the most common causes of discomfort following a reduction (**Fig. 12**).

Following reduction and splinting of the affected wrist, patients should have a repeat neurovascular examination and repeat plain radiographs of the wrist to assess the quality of the reduction. On discharge, patients should be referred to an orthopedic surgeon within days (preferably within 1 week) following the injury to evaluate for operative intervention. They should be instructed to loosen the ace wrap if the swelling and pain worsens. However, a return to the ED should

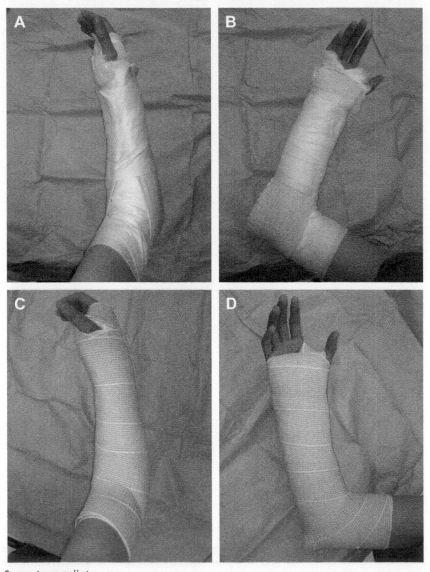

Fig. 9. (*A–D*) Sugar-tong splint.

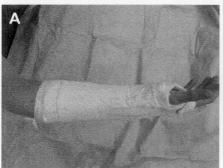
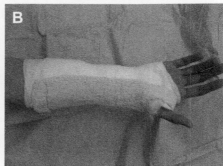

Fig. 10. (*A, B*) Radial gutter splint.

also be instructed if they develop worsening pain in the hand and wrist, numbness or tingling in the fingers, weakness of the hand and fingers, or if the fingers become progressively pale or cyanotic.[35,60] This is often a result of splinting and ace wrapping applied too tightly and can be rectified by loosening of the wrap and monitoring for return of neurologic function.[60] If a patient returns with this presentation, the splint should be removed. If symptoms persist, emergent orthopedic evaluation is indicated.

SURGICAL INDICATIONS

Even in cases where the practitioner in the ED initially evaluating and treating the patient for a distal radius fracture will not be ultimately providing definitive treatment, it remains valuable to understand the surgical indications for distal radius fractures to better communicate with the patient and facilitate specialty consultation. Outpatient surgical indications are ultimately based on a variety of factors including patient demographics, age, concomitant injuries, fracture alignment, and fracture stability.

Regarding fracture alignment, acceptable parameters following closed reduction include a residual radial inclination greater than or equal to 15 degrees on posteroanterior view, volar tilt less than 20 degrees dorsally on the lateral view, radial length of less than or equal to 5 mm of shortening on the posteroanterior view, and articular incongruity of less than 2 mm of step-off for intra-articular fractures. If these parameters are met following closed reduction, nonoperative management has a higher likelihood of successful outcome. These are not absolute parameters for operative versus nonoperative management, and can be titrated up and down depending on the patient's age and demands. Moreover, all fractures that are adequately reduced initially are not necessarily stable and may lose reduction with nonoperative management. Radiographic parameters suggestive of instability are dorsal comminution that is greater than half of the width laterally, an initial dorsal tilt greater than 20 degrees, initial fragment translation greater than 1 cm, initial radial shortening more than 5 mm, intra-articular disruption, associated ulna fractures, volar metaphyseal comminution, or severe osteoporosis.

Associated injuries may change operative indications. Open fractures or acute carpal tunnel syndromes necessitate early operative intervention. Additionally, multiply injured patients with bilateral distal radius fractures, concomitant ipsilateral or bilateral upper extremity fractures, or ipsilateral carpal injuries may also require operative intervention.

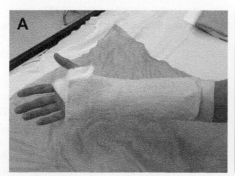
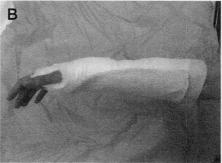

Fig. 11. (*A, B*) Volar splint.

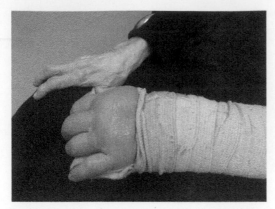

Fig. 12. Example of an ace wrap applied too tight and inappropriately. The patient presents 3 days after ED fracture reduction and splinting of her distal radius fracture. The wrap should be applied proximally to distally, include the base of the hand, and not be too tight. If applied too tight, excessive hand swelling and pain can ensue, as in this case.

Ultimately, the final decision of the need for operative intervention does not need to be made immediately in the ED setting. However, these variables may allow the nonsurgical practitioner to offer guidance to the injured patient.

SUMMARY

Distal radius fractures are one of the most common fractures seen in the ED. Therefore, appropriate clinical recognition and management by all practitioners is important. Concomitant traumatic injuries must be appropriately worked-up. Findings potentially warranting urgent surgical intervention include open fractures, vascular injury, and acute carpal tunnel syndrome. Indications for fracture reduction in the ED include excessive deformity, any joint dislocation or subluxation, and dorsal tilt greater than 20 degrees. Fractures should be adequately reduced and diligently splinted as described before outpatient follow-up. Ace wrapping should be applied loosely and the patient should be instructed to loosen the dressing and/or return to the ED for increased pain or symptoms of neurovascular compromise. Finally, outpatient surgical indications are ultimately based on a variety of factors including patient demographics, age, concomitant injuries, fracture alignment, and fracture stability.

REFERENCES

1. De Lorenzo RA, Mayer D, Geehr EC. Analyzing clinical case distributions to improve an emergency medicine clerkship. Ann Emerg Med 1990;19(7): 746–51.

2. National Hospital Ambulatory Medical Care Survey: 2008 Emergency Department Summary Tables - 2008_ed_web_tables.pdf. Available at: http://www.cdc.gov/nchs/data/ahcd/nhamcs_emergency/2008_ed_web_tables.pdf. Accessed April 27, 2014.

3. Comer GC, Liang E, Bishop JA. Lack of proficiency in musculoskeletal medicine among emergency medicine physicians. J Orthop Trauma 2014;28(4):e85–7. http://dx.doi.org/10.1097/BOT.0b013e3182a66829.

4. Bernstein J, Garcia GH, Guevara JL, et al. Progress report: the prevalence of required medical school instruction in musculoskeletal medicine at decade's end. Clin Orthop 2011;469(3):895–7. http://dx.doi.org/10.1007/s11999-010-1477-3.

5. Day CS, Yeh AC, Franko O, et al. Musculoskeletal medicine: an assessment of the attitudes and knowledge of medical students at Harvard Medical School. Acad Med 2007;82(5):452–7. http://dx.doi.org/10.1097/ACM.0b013e31803ea860.

6. Freedman KB, Bernstein J. Educational deficiencies in musculoskeletal medicine. J Bone Joint Surg Am 2002;84A(4):604–8.

7. Day CS, Yeh AC. Evidence of educational inadequacies in region-specific musculoskeletal medicine. Clin Orthop 2008;466(10):2542–7. http://dx.doi.org/10.1007/s11999-008-0379-0.

8. Schmale GA. More evidence of educational inadequacies in musculoskeletal medicine. Clin Orthop 2005;437:251–9.

9. Shauver MJ, Clapham PJ, Chung KC. An economic analysis of outcomes and complications of treating distal radius fractures in the elderly. J Hand Surg 2011;36(12):1912–8.e1-3. http://dx.doi.org/10.1016/j.jhsa.2011.09.039.

10. Baron JA, Karagas M, Barrett J, et al. Basic epidemiology of fractures of the upper and lower limb among Americans over 65 years of age. Epidemiology 1996;7(6):612–8.

11. Court-Brown CM, Caesar B. Epidemiology of adult fractures: a review. Injury 2006;37(8):691–7. http://dx.doi.org/10.1016/j.injury.2006.04.130.

12. Chung KC, Spilson SV. The frequency and epidemiology of hand and forearm fractures in the United States. J Hand Surg 2001;26(5):908–15. http://dx.doi.org/10.1053/jhsu.2001.26322.

13. Nellans KW, Kowalski E, Chung KC. The epidemiology of distal radius fractures. Hand Clin 2012;28(2):113–25. http://dx.doi.org/10.1016/j.hcl.2012.02.001.

14. Chung KC, Shauver MJ, Yin H, et al. Variations in the use of internal fixation for distal radial fracture in the United States Medicare population. J Bone Joint Surg Am 2011;93(23):2154–62. http://dx.doi.org/10.2106/JBJS.J.012802.

15. Ray NF, Chan JK, Thamer M, et al. Medical expenditures for the treatment of osteoporotic fractures in the United States in 1995: report from the National

Osteoporosis Foundation. J Bone Miner Res 1997;
12(1):24–35.   http://dx.doi.org/10.1359/jbmr.1997.
12.1.24.

16. Melton LJ III, Amadio PC, Crowson CS, et al. Long-
term trends in the incidence of distal forearm fractures. Osteoporos Int 1998;8(4):341–8.

17. De Putter CE, van Beeck EF, Looman CW, et al.
Trends in wrist fractures in children and adolescents,
1997-2009. J Hand Surg Am 2011;36(11):1810–5.
e2. http://dx.doi.org/10.1016/j.jhsa.2011.08.006.

18. Hagino H, Yamamoto K, Ohshiro H, et al. Changing
incidence of hip, distal radius, and proximal humerus fractures in Tottori Prefecture, Japan. Bone 1999;
24(3):265–70.

19. Thompson PW, Taylor J, Dawson A. The annual incidence and seasonal variation of fractures of the
distal radius in men and women over 25 years in
Dorset, UK. Injury 2004;35(5):462–6. http://dx.doi.
org/10.1016/S0020-1383(03)00117-7.

20. Brenner H, Arndt V. Epidemiology in aging research.
Exp Gerontol 2004;39(5):679–86. http://dx.doi.org/
10.1016/j.exger.2004.02.006.

21. Schoenborn CA. Health habits of U.S. adults, 1985:
the "Alameda 7" revisited. Public Health Rep 1986;
101(6):571–80.

22. Ring D, Jupiter JB. Treatment of osteoporotic distal
radius fractures. Osteoporos Int 2005;16(Suppl 2):
S80–4. http://dx.doi.org/10.1007/s00198-004-1808-x.

23. Rowe JW, Kahn RL. Successful aging. New York:
Pantheon Books; 1998. Available at: https://con-
nect.tjuh.org/dana-na/auth/url_11/welcome.cgi. Accessed May 4, 2014.

24. Cummings SR, Black DM, Rubin SM. Lifetime risks
of hip, Colles', or vertebral fracture and coronary
heart disease among white postmenopausal
women. Arch Intern Med 1989;149(11):2445–8.

25. Singer BR, McLauchlan GJ, Robinson CM, et al.
Epidemiology of fractures in 15,000 adults: the influence of age and gender. J Bone Joint Surg Br 1998;
80(2):243–8.

26. Kanterewicz E, Yañez A, Pérez-Pons A, et al. Association between Colles' fracture and low bone
mass: age-based differences in postmenopausal
women. Osteoporos Int 2002;13(10):824–8. http://
dx.doi.org/10.1007/s001980200114.

27. Löfman O, Hallberg I, Berglund K, et al. Women with
low-energy fracture should be investigated for osteoporosis. Acta Orthop 2007;78(6):813–21. http://dx.
doi.org/10.1080/17453670710014608.

28. Øyen J, Rohde GE, Hochberg M, et al. Low-energy distal radius fractures in middle-aged and
elderly women-seasonal variations, prevalence of
osteoporosis, and associates with fractures. Osteoporos Int 2010;21(7):1247–55. http://dx.doi.org/10.
1007/s00198-009-1065-0.

29. Oyen J, Brudvik C, Gjesdal CG, et al. Osteoporosis
as a risk factor for distal radial fractures: a case-

control study. J Bone Joint Surg Am 2011;93(4):
348–56. http://dx.doi.org/10.2106/JBJS.J.00303.

30. Øyen J, Rohde G, Hochberg M, et al. Low bone min-
eral density is a significant risk factor for low-energy
distal radius fractures in middle-aged and elderly
men: a case-control study. BMC Musculoskelet Disord 2011;12:67. http://dx.doi.org/10.1186/1471-
2474-12-67.

31. Zalavras CG, Patzakis MJ. Open fractures: evaluation and management. J Am Acad Orthop Surg
2003;11(3):212–9.

32. Gustilo RB, Anderson JT. Prevention of infection in
the treatment of one thousand and twenty-five
open fractures of long bones: retrospective and prospective analyses. J Bone Joint Surg Am 1976;
58(4):453–8.

33. Patzakis MJ, Wilkins J. Factors influencing infection
rate in open fracture wounds. Clin Orthop 1989;
243:36–40.

34. Cleland JA, Koppenhaver S. Netter's orthopaedic clinical examination: an evidence-based approach. 2nd
edition. Philadelphia (PA): Saunders Elsevier; 2011.

35. Hammert WC, Calfee RP, Bozentka DJ, et al. ASSH:
manual of hand surgery. Philadelphia (PA): Lippincott Williams & Wilkins; 2010.

36. Sponsel KH, Palm ET. Carpal tunnel syndrome
following Colles' fracture. Surg Gynecol Obstet
1965;121(6):1252–6.

37. Niver GE, Ilyas AM. Carpal tunnel syndrome after
distal radius fracture. Orthop Clin North Am 2012;
43(4):521–7. http://dx.doi.org/10.1016/j.ocl.2012.
07.021.

38. Gelberman RH, Garfin SR, Hergenroeder PT, et al.
Compartment syndromes of the forearm: diagnosis
and treatment. Clin Orthop 1981;161:252–61.

39. Adamson JE, Srouji SJ, Horton CE, et al. The acute
carpal tunnel syndrome. Plast Reconstr Surg 1971;
47(4):332–6.

40. Bauman TD, Gelberman RH, Mubarak SJ, et al. The
acute carpal tunnel syndrome. Clin Orthop
1981;(156):151–6.

41. Lewis MH. Median nerve decompression after Colles's
fracture. J Bone Joint Surg Br 1978;60B(2):195–6.

42. Medoff RJ. Essential radiographic evaluation
for distal radius fractures. Hand Clin 2005;21(3):
279–88. http://dx.doi.org/10.1016/j.hcl.2005.02.008.

43. Szabo RM. Distal radioulnar joint instability. J Bone
Joint Surg Am 2006;88(4):884–94.

44. Harness NG, Ring D, Zurakowski D, et al. The influence of three-dimensional computed tomography
reconstructions on the characterization and treatment of distal radial fractures. J Bone Joint Surg
Am 2006;88(6):1315–23. http://dx.doi.org/10.2106/
JBJS.E.00686.

45. Knirk JL, Jupiter JB. Intra-articular fractures of the
distal end of the radius in young adults. J Bone Joint
Surg Am 1986;68(5):647–59.

46. Bleck TP. *Clostridum tetani* (Tetanus). In: Mandell G, Douglas R, Bennett J, editors. Principles and practice of infectious diseases. 6th edition. Philadelphia: Churchill Livingstone; 2005. p. 1289–312.

47. Patzakis MJ, Wilkins J, Moore TM. Considerations in reducing the infection rate in open tibial fractures. Clin Orthop 1983;178:36–41.

48. Cross WW, Swiontkowski MF. Treatment principles in the management of open fractures. Indian J Orthop 2008;42(4):377–86.

49. Crowley DJ, Kanakaris NK, Giannoudis PV. Debridement and wound closure of open fractures: the impact of the time factor on infection rates. Injury 2007;38(8):879–89.

50. Zumsteg JW, Molina CS, Lee DH, et al. Factors influencing infection rates after open fractures of the radius and/or ulna. J Hand Surg 2014;39(5):956–61.

51. Rozental TD, Beredjiklian PK, Steinberg DR, et al. Open fractures of the distal radius. J Hand Surg 2002;27(1):77–85.

52. Myderrizi N, Mema B. The hematoma block an effective alternative for fracture reduction in distal radius fractures. Med Arh 2011;65(4):239–42.

53. Blichert-Toft M, Jensen HK. Colles' fracture treated with modified Böhler technique. Acta Orthop Scand 1971;42(1):45–57.

54. Case RD. Haematoma block: a safe method of reducing Colles' fractures. Injury 1985;16(7):469–70.

55. Liles R, Frierson JN, Wolf CL, et al. Reduction of Colles' fracture by weight traction under local anesthesia. South Med J 1969;62(1):45–8.

56. Earnshaw SA, Aladin A, Surendran S, et al. Closed reduction of Colles fractures: comparison of manual manipulation and finger-trap traction: a prospective, randomized study. J Bone Joint Surg Am 2002; 84A(3):354–8.

57. Agee JM. Distal radius fractures. Multiplanar ligamentotaxis. Hand Clin 1993;9(4):577–85.

58. Bong MR, Egol KA, Leibman M, et al. A comparison of immediate postreduction splinting constructs for controlling initial displacement of fractures of the distal radius: a prospective randomized study of long-arm versus short-arm splinting. J Hand Surg 2006;31(5):766–70. http://dx.doi.org/10.1016/j.jhsa. 2006.01.016.

59. Egol KA, Koval KJ, Zuckerman JD. Handbook of fractures. 4th edition. Lippincott Williams & Wilkins; 2010.

60. Halanski M, Noonan KJ. Cast and splint immobilization: complications. J Am Acad Orthop Surg 2008; 16(1):30–40.

The Management of Acute and Chronic Elbow Instability

Irfan Ahmed, MD[a],*, Jaydev Mistry, BS[b]

KEYWORDS

- Elbow dislocation • Instability • Collateral ligaments • Elbow joint injuries
- Posterolateral rotatory instability

KEY POINTS

- "Elbow instability" includes a wide variety of disorders from simple acute dislocations to complex dislocations with concomitant injuries to osseous and ligamentous structures.
- Simple dislocations are the most common and can usually be treated with closed reduction and early active motion to produce excellent outcomes.
- Complex elbow dislocations generally require surgical intervention to repair the soft tissue and associated fractures to yield stability and facilitate early active motion.
- Residual instability may require dynamic bracing or ligament reconstruction depending on the extent of ligamentous deficiency.
- Chronic elbow dislocations require open reduction and hinged external fixation versus static bridging temporary internal fixation to restore stability.

ACUTE AND CHRONIC ELBOW INSTABILITY

The elbow is the second most commonly dislocated major joint in adults. It is also the most commonly dislocated major joint in the pediatric population, with dislocations accounting for 10% to 25% of all elbow injuries.[1] The mean age is 30 years and it is more common in males.

Instability of the elbow can range from simple dislocation with no associated fractures to more complex patterns with varying degrees of bony and ligamentous injuries. Chronic instability can present with recurrent subluxation or dislocation owing to incompetence of the lateral ulnar collateral ligament (LUCL).

Understanding elbow instability requires a thorough knowledge of the articular elements, anatomy of the lateral collateral ligament complex, and the mechanism of elbow subluxation and dislocation.

Anatomy

The elbow is a trochoginglymoid joint with 2 principle arcs of motion: flexion–extension and pronation–supination. The ulnohumeral articulation contributes primarily to flexion–extension with pronation–supination occurring through the radiohumeral articulation. The elbow is not a true hinge and simulated motion studies suggest that there are 3° to 4° of potential varus and valgus laxity and axial laxity that may occur through the range of motion of the joint,[2] but for practical purposes it can be considered to move as a uniaxial articulation, except at extremes of range. The axis of rotation passes through the center of the arcs formed by the sulcus of the trochlea and the capitellum.[3]

The elbow is a highly congruent joint and thus has a high degree of inherent stability. The osseous anatomy of the distal humerus and

a Department of Orthopedics, Rutgers University Hospital, New Jersey Medical School, 140 Bergen Street, ACC D1610, Newark, NJ 07103, USA; b Rutgers University Hospital, New Jersey Medical School, 140 Bergen Street, ACCD1610, Newark, NJ 07103, USA
* Corresponding author.
E-mail address: ahmedi2@njms.rutgers.edu

Orthop Clin N Am 46 (2015) 271–280
http://dx.doi.org/10.1016/j.ocl.2014.11.008
0030-5898/15/$ – see front matter Published by Elsevier Inc.

proximal ulna provide most of the inherent stability of the elbow. This stability is based on both static and dynamic constraints. Static restraints are primarily the ulnohumeral articulation, the medial collateral ligament (MCL) and the lateral collateral ligament (LCL), specifically the ulnar part of the LCL. Other static restraints include the radial head, the common flexor and extensor origins, and the capsule.

The major determinant of stability, however, is the ulnohumeral joint, specifically the coronoid. The coronoid process, which consists of a tip, body, anterolateral facet, and anteromedial facet, acts as an anterior buttress, resisting the posteriorly directed forces from the triceps, brachioradialis, or the biceps acting at the elbow joint,[4] resisting subluxation in both flexion and extension. Its role in preventing posteromedial rotatory instability of the elbow has also been described.[5] Interlocking of the coronoid and olecranon processes provides added ulnohumeral stability at extremes of motion. Clinical evidence suggests that at least 50% of the coronoid must be present for the ulnohumeral joint to be functional.[6] Absence of the radial head further and dramatically compromises the elbow with a 50% or greater coronoid deficiency. The radial head should not be removed from a dislocated elbow in which the coronoid is fractured, unless the coronoid and ligaments can be repaired reliably.

The radial head may contribute up to 30% of the stability of the elbow against a valgus stress, and up to 75% with disruption of the MCL complex,[7] where it becomes the primary restraint to valgus stress.

Dynamic stabilizers include muscles crossing the elbow joint that produce compressive forces at the articulation. The muscles contributing most to this stability are the anconeus, triceps, and brachialis. The anconeus originates near the lateral epicondyle, has a broad, fan-shaped insertion on the ulna, and serves as a major dynamic stabilizer of the elbow, preventing posterolateral rotational displacement.

The medial collateral ligament and lateral collateral ligament complexes, in combination with the anterior capsule, the posterior capsule, and the ulnohumeral articulation, provide important static restraints to elbow instability. The medial collateral ligament is composed of the anterior oblique ligament, the posterior oblique ligament, and the transverse ligament. The strongest and most crucial structure of this segment is the anterior oblique ligament (**Fig. 1**), because it is the primary restraint to applied valgus force in conjunction with the radial head. Studies have demonstrated that as long as there is an intact anterior oblique

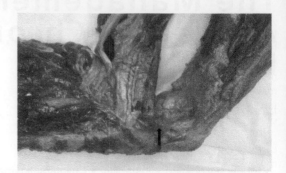

Fig. 1. Cadaver model showing medial view of elbow and anterior band of medial collateral ligament (*black arrow*).

ligament, there is minimal change in joint stability, even in the absence of an incompetent radial head. In contrast, anterior oblique ligament release combined with excised radial head results in gross instability of the elbow joint.[8,9]

The lateral collateral ligament complex consists of the radial collateral ligament, the LUCL, and the annular ligament. The radial collateral ligament originates from the lateral epicondyle and terminates by blending into the annular ligament. As a unit, it serves to stabilize the proximal radioulnar joint. The LUCL (**Fig. 2**), originating from the lateral epicondyle, blends with the fibers from the annular ligament, but arches superficially and distal to it. The LUCL functions as the primary restraint to varus stress and is impaired in posterolateral rotatory instability of the joint.[10]

The anterior capsule of the elbow is thin, but provides a significant stabilizing effect when it is taut in extension, although that decreases as the elbow approaches 90° of flexion. Anteriorly, the capsule attaches to the anterior region of the sigmoid notch as well as the proximal aspect of the olecranon fossa. This capsule has been found to commonly be torn in elbow dislocations.[10]

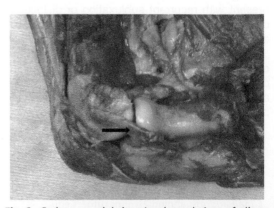

Fig. 2. Cadaver model showing lateral view of elbow with lateral ulnar collateral ligament (*black arrow*).

The thin posterior capsule, composed mainly of transverse fibers, stretches across the olecranon fossae to form a transverse band. On the ulnar aspect of the elbow, the capsule forms the posterior portion of the annular ligament. The attachment of the posterior capsule to the triceps tendon prevents the capsule from getting caught during extension.[10]

The muscles forming the medial complex of the elbow include the flexor carpi ulnaris, flexor carpi radialis, flexor digitorum superficialis, and pronator teres. Together, this group provides a support that is capable of resisting valgus forces. In comparison, the muscles forming the lateral complex of the elbow (extensor carpi ulnaris, extensor digitorum communis, extensor carpi radialis brevis, extensor carpi radialis longus, and anconeus) provide a reinforcement to resist varus forces. This has been found to be significant in cases of lateral collateral ligament deficiency. Together, the medial and lateral musculotendinous complexes contribute to a dynamic stability of the elbow as a result of compression of the joint surfaces against each other.[8] As long as these remain constraints intact, namely the ulnohumeral articulation, lateral collateral ligament, and medial collateral ligament, the elbow will be stable.

Evaluation and Assessment

The most common types of elbow dislocations are those that occur posteriorly. Typically, dislocation refers to the displacement of the radius and ulna relative to the humerus. Some studies explain that dislocations occur most frequently occur as a result of a fall on an outstretched hand, whereas others describe them occurring most commonly from athletic injuries.[11] Either way, instability can be classified by the direction of instability, the presence or absence of fractures (complex vs simple, respectively), and whether they are acute or chronic in nature.[12]

First, however, assessment of elbow instability must be performed owing to the potential high-energy trauma typically associated with elbow dislocations. Obtaining the history should allow one to discern the mechanism of injury, severity of injury, and additional morbidities. After the life- and limb-threatening injuries have been treated, the physical examination should focus on the involved limb. The injured elbow should be assessed for deformities and presence of open injury. A dislocated elbow often appears with the forearm held in varus and supination. Before any manipulation, assessment of neurovascular status should be determined. In particular, entrapment of the brachial artery, median nerve, and ulnar nerve are of concern owing to their increased frequency of injury during manipulation.[13] Associated injuries should be sought out with evaluation of the ipsilateral shoulder and wrist, along with the ipsilateral distal radial–ulnar joint and interosseous membrane. Localized swelling owing to soft tissue disruption is common, and may lead to constriction of the associated fascial compartments, resulting in increased intracompartmental pressures. As such, all patients presenting with an acute dislocation should be initially evaluated for the presence and development of compartment syndrome.[14,15]

Simple Dislocation

Simple dislocations most commonly occur in a posterior and lateral manner without major fracture (**Fig. 3**). Ten percent of cases, however, can have a minor avulsion near the epicondyles and/or coronoid process; however, they are not significant.[12]

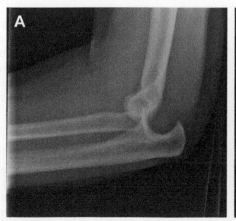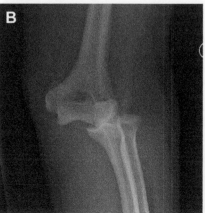

Fig. 3. (A) Lateral and (B) anteroposterior radiographs of a simple elbow dislocation. Note disruption of the ulnohumeral and radiocapitellar joints, without a major fracture of the coronoid and the radial head.

Anterior dislocations, although uncommon, should remain in the differential diagnosis owing to their association with triceps disruption or olecranon fractures. It should also be noted that the even more rare divergent dislocation is typically associated with high-energy trauma. The mechanism of a posterior dislocation is typically a combination of valgus, supination, or external rotation of the forearm, causing an axial load through the elbow.[14] The summation of these forces initiates a sequence of soft tissue injuries from the lateral to medial aspects of the elbow, leading to posterolateral rotation of the forearm relative to the humerus culminating in posterior dislocation of the proximal radius and ulna as the coronoid is displaced posteriorly in relation to the trochlea[16–18] and can be clinically reproduced by a maneuver known as the "lateral pivot shift test,"[19] which is discussed elsewhere in this article. The resulting tissue disruption has been classified into 3 stages.[15,20]

Stage 1 is characterized by partial or complete disruption of the lateral collateral ligament with complete disruption of the ulnar component. The resulting posterolateral subluxation may be reduced spontaneously. In the event of further anterior and posterior capsular disruption, a *stage 2* dislocation may occur with the coronoid in a "perched" position on the humeral trochlea; in essence, the coronoid has not slipped behind the trochlea (**Fig. 4**).[21] This is also known as an incomplete subluxation, and is possible with disruption of the lateral collateral ligament with some maintenance of the medial collateral ligament.[16] A *stage 3* dislocation occurs after persistent force has been applied, disrupting the MCL and causing a

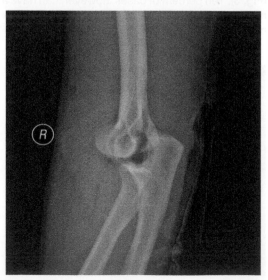

Fig. 4. Lateral radiograph demonstrating "Perched" or stage 2 elbow dislocation.

posterior dislocation. This stage has been subdivided into parts.[9] *Stage 3A* is characterized by disruption of all the soft tissues around to and including the posterior part of the medial collateral ligament. The anterior band of the medial collateral ligament is intact, allowing for posterior dislocation and pivoting of the elbow around the band. Reduction is completed by manipulation of the elbow while in supination and valgus, which mimics the deformity. In *stage 3B*, the entire medial collateral complex is disturbed; however, after reduction, valgus, varus, and rotatory instability are still present. *Stage 3C* is characterized by complete stripping of soft tissues around the distal humerus, resulting in an instability so severe that the elbow is capable of dislocation or subluxation, even in a cast set to flexion of 90°. The most effective reduction is maintained typically by flexion of the elbow past 90° to 110°. In addition to the ligamentous compromise in stage 3C dislocation, the origin of forearm flexor and pronator muscles (which are secondary dynamic stabilizers of the elbow) is compromised.

The primary objective of treatment for a simple dislocation is to provide a stable reduction that allows for early active range of motion. The reduction can be completed with or without sedation.[10] The reduction is performed by flexing the elbow to approximately 25° while applying longitudinal traction combined with supination at the forearm and countertraction at the upper arm provided by an assistant.[1,12] Valgus and varus instability should be assessed with the elbow in 30° of flexion and full extension. Initial management includes immobilization for approximately 2 to 3 weeks, followed by flexion and extension in a hinged splint for 4 weeks. Afterward, unrestricted flexion and extension may be allowed; however, care should be taken to avoid excessive valgus load. Development of a significant flexion contracture is uncommon in this injury.[21]

After complete dislocations, some instability will be present, given that both medial and lateral ligaments have been disturbed. If dislocation occurs during extension, the elbow should be reassessed with the forearm in pronation. If this position proves to be more stable, a hinged brace should be applied with the forearm placed in pronation. It should be noted that, if greater than 45° of pronation are required to maintain the reduction, operative intervention is indicated.[1,12,20,22,23]

In the event of surgery, a midline posterior approach is used, although medial and lateral approaches may also be used, depending on surgeon preference. A posterior approach allows for raising fasciocutaneous flaps enabling circumferential access,[24] as well as minimal disruption of local cutaneous nerves. In contrast with lateral and medial incision sites, fewer cutaneous nerves cross in the posterior midline.[25] It is absolutely critical that the ulnar nerve be identified and protected, and transposed anteriorly if necessary. This is standard during any repair procedures involving the medial compartment of the elbow. Complete dislocations almost always include disruption of the medial collateral ligament complex,[18,26–28] sometimes even avulsing the overlying flexor–pronator muscular structures.[26–28] On the opposite side, avulsion of the common extensor origin on the lateral epicondyle can aid in exposing the lateral collateral ligament complex.[26,29] In both cases, the ligamentous complexes can be repaired with large, braided, nonabsorbable sutures, suture anchors, bone tunnels, or in certain chronic situations autogenous tendon grafts. After surgery, the stability of the elbow must be assessed. If instability persists, a hinged external fixator with skeletal fixation should be applied. This can ensure joint range of motion with maintenance of joint reduction.[11,24] If the joint is stable after surgery, a hinged brace with our without an extension block can be used for 4 to 6 weeks. In addition to a supervised range-of-motion program, follow-up radiographs should be obtained to ensure that the joint is maintained in appropriate reduction.[14]

Complex Fracture–Dislocation

Appropriately termed the "terrible triad," the combination of ligamentous injury with coronoid and radial head fractures (**Fig. 5**) has been found to have a high complication rate.[30] The most effective method to stabilize these injuries requires surgical intervention to allow for return to early motion. Closed reduction often results in redislocation, which may risk further damage. This type of injury can be appropriately assessed with 3-dimensional CT reconstructions to help

address each component of the injury. Goals of surgery include restoration of the anterior bony buttress, which consists of the coronoid process and radial head, and repair of the medial collateral ligament and the LUCL. Even small coronoid fractures should be repaired, if possible, because the repair adds an additional reinforcement against dislocation and restoration of function of the anterior capsule.[31] The coronoid can be secured with a combination of suture fixation and/or screw fixation. After repair or replacement of the radial head, the radial extensor mass and lateral collateral ligament can be reattached to the lateral condyle of the humerus (**Fig. 6**). This is immediately followed by an assessment of stability through a full range of motion. If there is redislocation during elbow extension before reaching 30° to 40° from full extension, it may be necessary to repair the medial collateral ligament and apply a hinged external fixator.[32,33] If redislocation occurs before the elbow approaches full extension, it will likely also be unstable in a cast or splint.[34]

Chronic Posterolateral Rotatory Instability

Although many structures are disrupted in an elbow dislocation, chronic instability is primarily owing to a deficiency in the lateral collateral ligament resulting in posterolateral rotatory instability. Some studies have reported that nearly one-third of patients with a simple dislocation of the elbow treated by closed reduction had long-term symptoms of instability.[35] Often, these patients present with a history of persistent, recurring pain, and clicking, catching, or subluxation within the range of motion. Patients generally recall 1 episode of trauma that may or may not have resulted in a dislocation, or sometimes even iatrogenic cause, such as an excessively lateral surgical approach as in the release of lateral epicondylitis, can result in posterolateral instability.

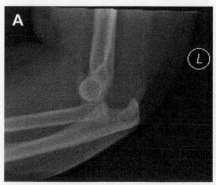
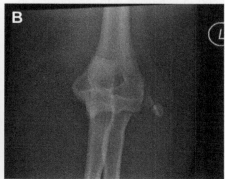

Fig. 5. (*A*) Lateral and (*B*) anteroposterior radiographs of a complex fracture-dislocation Lateral x-ray. Note fracture of both the radial head and coronoid consist with a terrible triad injury.

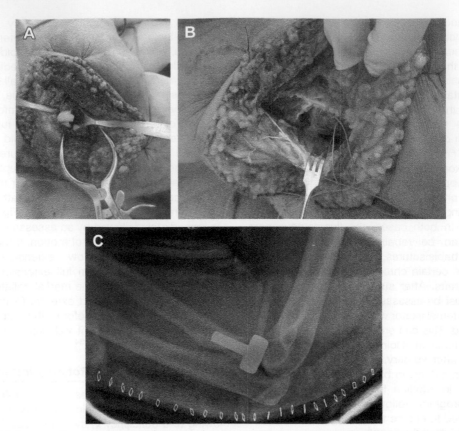

Fig. 6. (*A*) Intraoperative view showing fracture of radial head in an acute complex elbow dislocation. (*B*) Radial head has been surgically resected. Note the bare lateral condyle of humerus with a suture anchor placed indicating the site of traumatic avulsion of the lateral collateral ligament origin. (*C*) Postoperative lateral radiograph demonstrating radial head replacement with a reduced and concentric elbow joint.

Range of motion in these patients is usually pain free, with negative valgus and varus stress testing. The "lateral pivot shift test" is the most sensitive test for clinical diagnosis of posterolateral rotatory instability, and is often performed under general anesthesia (**Fig. 7**).[36] To recreate the mechanism of instability, the patient lays supine on the examination table and has the involved arm overhead with the shoulder in external rotation. Next, the elbow is placed in extension with the forearm in supination while a valgus load is simultaneously applied. The elbow is then slowly brought from extension into flexion, and the radial head is felt to slip back in place.[19,30] The test is positive if a visible or palpable clunk is elicited. Even simpler, the patient can be asked to push up from a chair with their forearms in supination. If pain or instability is felt as the elbow proceeds to extension, the test is positive.[36] Another test known as the posterolateral rotatory drawer test has the elbow placed in 40° to 90° of flexion while applying an anteroposterior force on the radius and ulna. This is done to subluxate the forearm away from the humerus on the lateral side. The test is considered positive if subluxation or apprehension is elicited.[37]

Generally, plain radiographs are normal, but sometimes can show avulsion from the lateral epicondyle or widening and/or incongruency of the joint space between the radius and capitellum.[10]

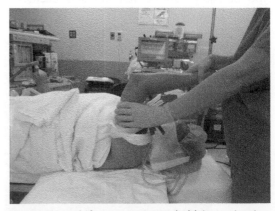

Fig. 7. Pivot shift test. Forearm held in supination, valgus load applied, and elbow brought from extension into flexion.

Stress radiographs or fluoroscopy can also be useful. When the lateral pivot shift test is performed, the elbow is placed in maximal rotatory subluxation and the ulnohumeral joint space is seen to be widened on lateral and anteroposterior views. Additionally, the lateral view can show posterior subluxation of the radial head.[10,19,30,36] If necessary, MR arthrography and diagnostic elbow arthroscopy can be used to visualize damage to the LCL complex and radial head subluxation, respectively.[10]

Generally, patients with less severe symptoms can be managed with extensor strengthening exercises or athletic neoprene sleeves, whereas patients with more severe symptoms and signs of chronic instability require surgery.[30] Patients requiring an operation often need reconstruction of the LUCL, usually with an autograft or allograft tendon. Various operative techniques successfully using different tendon graft sites have been investigated in the literature, including the palmaris longus, plantaris, gracilis, and semitendinosus.[36]

Chronic Elbow Dislocation

A chronic elbow dislocation is a disabling condition associated with severe limitation of elbow function and often significant pain. Neglected elbow dislocations or inadequate assessment after an attempted reduction can lead to a chronic dislocation of the elbow. Arthritic changes occur rapidly if the elbow is not reduced. Radiographs can readily make the diagnosis (**Fig. 8**); however, CT evaluation should be considered to help with surgical planning. The goals of treatment can be conflicting, because it involves restoring both a stable concentric joint while also facilitating early motion within a satisfactory arc of motion. In the younger population, treatment options vary depending on the degree of posttraumatic arthritis

present. If there is mild to moderate arthritis, then open reduction, reconstruction of medial and lateral collateral ligaments, and placement of a hinged external fixator is an option. There is a risk of redislocation, even with hinged external fixation (**Fig. 9**), and a temporary internal plate may be needed to keep the joint concentrically reduced albeit at the expense of total joint motion (**Fig. 10**). If there is more severe arthritis, distraction interpositional arthroplasty, or joint fusion may be considered. In the older age group, total elbow arthroplasty is also a good potential option.

Complications

Nerve and vessel injury

Approximately 20% of dislocations are complicated by a nerve injury, the most common being that of the ulnar nerve. This is generally owing to a valgus stretching of the nerve.[38] Median nerve involvement occurs secondary to stretch injuries or as a result of compression from swelling. The most common symptom is a transient paresthesia. However, a permanent deficit may result if the nerve is entrapped within the joint. Nerve entrapment can be potentially detected by MRI.[39]

Injuries to the brachial artery can include spasm, thrombosis, intimal damage, or rupture. Because these do not necessarily occur exclusively with neurologic symptoms, aggressive investigation and treatment of suspected injuries should be undertaken, including imaging, arterial reconstruction, stabilization of the joint, and even fasciotomy.

Chronic instability

Chronic instability is challenging to manage because it can be owing to a manifestation of many disruptions. It may be related to bony malunion or nonunion, bone loss, attenuation of ligamentous complexes, or even a combination

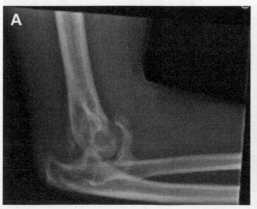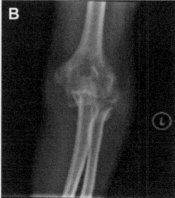

Fig. 8. (*A*) Lateral and (*B*) anteroposterior radiographs demonstrating a chronic elbow dislocation. Note the presence of surrounding heterotopic ossification.

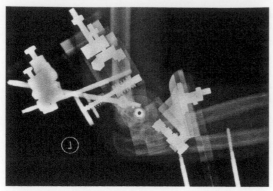

Fig. 9. Two weeks after open joint reduction, ligament reconstruction, and hinged external fixator placement of a chronic elbow dislocation, demonstrating residual subluxation of the elbow joint.

thereof. Up to 50% of patients can have laxity without demonstrating symptoms of frank ligamentous instability.[14] Deficiency in the lateral collateral ligament can result in an unsupported lateral forearm, which may cause rotation posterior to the humerus.[19] A symptomatic laxity can result in chronic instability, and therefore indicating ligament reconstruction.

Arthrosis/articular injury
As the initial injury becomes more complex, chondral damage from the initial injury may develop into more chronic problems. Even in the absence of radiographic evidence of fracture, osteochondral injury can readily occur after the elbow is

dislocated. Moreover, osteochondral fragments entrapped within the intra-articular joint space can result in further articular injury and may prompt surgical excision after closed reduction. This osteochondral injury can have an effect on the long-term functional outcomes of the joint.[40]

Compartment syndrome
Intracompartmental pressures can dramatically rise within the flexor compartment owing to intramuscular bleeding and edema, even in the absence of vascular injury. High clinical suspicion for compartment syndrome should be maintained with physical examination findings of pain on passive movement of the fingers and wrist, as well as pain out of proportion.[14]

Contracture/stiffness
Thickening and fibrosis of the anterior joint capsule is a common complication of both simple and complex elbow dislocations.[33] Greater loss of motion can occur in cases of complex elbow dislocation. Loss of motion can be minimized by prompt concentric reduction and institution of early motion. Bracing and physical therapy are acceptable treatments of an established contracture within 1 year of the injury. In the event that the contracture results in an arc of motion less than 30° to 130° that is unresponsive to bracing and therapy, capsulectomy may be indicated.[10,11,15]

Heterotopic ossification
These ossifications can be seen 4 to 6 weeks after injury on plain radiographs, and are present in up

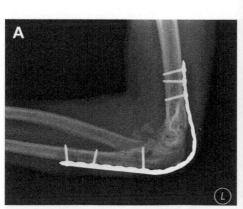

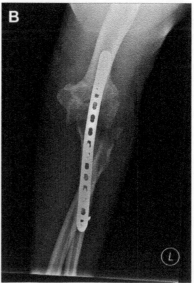

Fig. 10. (*A*) Lateral and (*B*) anteroposterior radiographs demonstrating a chronic elbow dislocation after an attempted open reduction and hinged external fixation, converted to a static temporary internal fixation with a bridge plate holding the elbow joint reduced. The hardware was removed and motion was started 4 weeks later.

to 75% of cases. Both the lateral and medial collateral ligaments are often involved; however, functional limitation is generally not observed. Fewer than 5% of cases involve motion-limiting ossification,[1] but it generally occurs within the anterior soft tissues. Risk factors such as patient age, gender, injury to central nervous system, and burns may play a role in the development of heterotopic ossification.[10] Gentle active and continuous passive motion reduces the risk of heterotopic ossification, whereas aggressive manipulation to combat stiffness results in an increased risk.[33] High-risk patients should be treated with heterotopic ossification prophylaxis such as low-dose radiation or nonsteroidal anti-inflammatory drug therapy. In the event of a motion-limiting ossification, resection should be undertaken 3 to 6 months after injury or once it has been determined that the ossification process has matured. This should be supported with the presence of a well-defined cortications of intralesional trabeculae on plain radiographs.[10,33]

SUMMARY

"Elbow instability" includes a wide variety of disorders ranging from simple acute dislocations to complex dislocations with additional injuries. These injuries require an assessment of the entire involved upper extremity with a full neurovascular examination. Simple dislocations are the most common and can usually be treated with closed reduction and early active motion to produce excellent outcomes. More complicated dislocations with fractures generally require operative intervention to repair the soft tissue and bony fragments to yield stability and early active motion. The presence of instability after closed reduction may require dynamic bracing or ligament reconstruction depending on the severity. Compromise of the LUCL causes posterolateral rotatory instability, the most common kind of recurrent instability. In these cases, conservative treatment is often unsuccessful and surgical reconstruction using tendon grafts is needed.

Overall, nonoperative treatment produces results that are equal to, if not better, than those of operative intervention. Flexion contracture, the most common complication, can be treated with early range-of-motion exercises. Recurrent instability is not a common complication; however, it generally requires surgical treatment. Chronic dislocations can be diagnosed with the lateral pivot-shift test, and although they can be initially managed conservatively, patients will likely require reconstruction of the LUCL using autograft or allograft tendon.

REFERENCES

1. Kuhn MA, Ross G. Acute elbow dislocations. Orthop Clin North Am 2008;39(2):155–61.
2. Tanaka S, An KN, Morrey BF. Kinematics and laxity of the ulnohumeral joint under valgus-varus stress. J Musculoskeletal Res 1998;2:45–54.
3. London JT. Kinematics of the elbow. J Bone Joint Surg Am 1981;63(4):529–35.
4. Morrey BF, O'Driscoll SW. Complex instability of the elbow. 3rd edition. Philadelphia: WB Saunders; 2000. p. 421–30.
5. O'Driscoll SW, Jupiter JB, Cohen MS, et al. Difficult elbow fractures: pearls and pitfalls. Instr Course Lect 2003;52:113–34.
6. Doornberg JN, van Duijn J, Ring D. Coronoid fracture height in terrible-triad injuries. J Hand Surg Am 2006;31(5):794–7.
7. An K, Morrey B. Biomechanics of the elbow. In: Morrey B, editor. The Elbow and its Disorders. 3rd edition. Philadelphia: WB Saunders; 2000. p. 43.
8. Safran MR, Baillargeon D. Soft-tissue stabilizers of the elbow. J Shoulder Elbow Surg 2005; 14(1 Suppl):179S–85S.
9. O'Driscoll SW. Elbow instability. Acta Orthop Belg 1999;65(4):404–15.
10. Modi CS, Lawrence E, Lawrence T. Elbow instability. Orthop Trauma 2012;26(5):316–27.
11. Cohen MS, Hastings H 2nd. Acute elbow dislocation: evaluation and management. J Am Acad Orthop Surg 1998;6(1):15–23.
12. Bell S. Elbow instability, mechanism and management. Curr Orthop 2008;22:90–103.
13. Hotchkiss R. Fractures and dislocation of the elbow. In: Rockwood C, Green DP, Bucholz RW, et al, editors. Rockwood and Green's fractures in adults, vol. 1. Philadelphia: Lippincott-Raven; 1996. p. 929–1025.
14. Sheps DM, Hildebrand KA, Boorman RS. Simple dislocations of the elbow: evaluation and treatment. Hand Clin 2004;20(4):389–404.
15. O'Driscoll SW. Elbow dislocations. In: Morrey BF, editor. The elbow and its disorders. 3rd edition. Philadelphia: WB Saunders; 2000. p. 409–20.
16. O'Driscoll SW, Morrey BF, Korinek S, et al. Elbow subluxation and dislocation. A spectrum of instability. Clin Orthop Relat Res 1992;(280):186–97.
17. Osborne G, Cotterill P. Recurrent dislocation of the elbow. J Bone Joint Surg Br 1966;48(2):340–6.
18. Sojbjerg JO, Helmig P, Kjaersgaard-Andersen P. Dislocation of the elbow: an experimental study of the ligamentous injuries. Orthopedics 1989;12(3): 461–3.
19. O'Driscoll SW, Bell DF, Morrey BF. Posterolateral rotatory instability of the elbow. J Bone Joint Surg Am 1991;73(3):440–6.
20. O'Driscoll SW, Jupiter JB, King GJ, et al. The unstable elbow. J Bone Joint Surg Am 2000;82:724–38.

21. Morrey BF. Acute and chronic instability of the elbow. J Am Acad Orthop Surg 1996;4(3):117–28.

22. Ebrahimzadeh MH, Amadzadeh-Chabock H, Ring D. Traumatic elbow instability. J Hand Surg Am 2010;35(7):1220–5.

23. Mudgal C, Jupiter J. New concepts in dislocation of the elbow. Tech Orthop 2008;23:142–57.

24. Hildebrand KA, Patterson SD, King GJ. Acute elbow dislocations: simple and complex. Orthop Clin North Am 1999;30(1):63–79.

25. Dowdy PA, Bain GI, King GJ, et al. The midline posterior elbow incision. An anatomical appraisal. J Bone Joint Surg Br 1995;77(5):696–9.

26. Josefsson PO, Johnell O, Wendeberg B. Ligamentous injuries in dislocations of the elbow joint. Clin Orthop Relat Res 1987;(221):221–5.

27. Josefsson PO, Gentz CF, Johnell O, et al. Surgical versus non-surgical treatment of ligamentous injuries following dislocation of the elbow joint. A prospective randomized study. J Bone Joint Surg Am 1987;69(4):605–8.

28. Josefsson PO, Gentz CF, Johnell O, et al. Surgical versus nonsurgical treatment of ligamentous injuries following dislocations of the elbow joint. Clin Orthop Relat Res 1987;(214):165–9.

29. McKee MD, Schemitsch EH, Sala MJ, et al. The pathoanatomy of lateral ligamentous disruption in complex elbow instability. J Shoulder Elbow Surg 2003;12(4):391–6.

30. Dyer G, Ring D. My approach to the terrible triad injury. Oper Tech Orthop 2010;20:11–6.

31. Ring D, Jupiter J. Operative fixation and reconstruction of the coronoid. Tech Orthop 2000;15.

32. Morrey B. Complex instability of the elbow. J Bone Joint Surg 1997;79A:460–9.

33. Ring D, Jupiter JB. Fracture-dislocation of the elbow. J Bone Joint Surg Am 1998;80(4):566–80.

34. Josefsson PO, Gentz CF, Johnell O, et al. Dislocations of the elbow and intraarticular fractures. Clin Orthop Relat Res 1989;(246):126–30.

35. Mehlhoff TL, Noble PC, Bennett JB, et al. Simply dislocation of the elbow in the adult. Results after closed treatment. J Bone Joint Surg 1998;70: 244–9.

36. Cheung EV. Chronic lateral elbow instability. Orthop Clin North Am 2008;39(2):221–8, vi–vii.

37. Phillips CS, Segalman KA. Diagnosis and treatment of post-traumatic medial and lateral elbow ligament incompetence. Hand Clin 2002;18(1):149–59.

38. Linscheid RL, Wheeler DK. Elbow dislocations. JAMA 1965;194(11):1171–6.

39. Akansel G, Dalbayrak S, Yilmaz M, et al. MRI demonstration of intra-articular median nerve entrapment after elbow dislocation. Skeletal Radiol 2003;32(9):537–41.

40. Durig M, Müller W, Rüedi TP, et al. The operative treatment of elbow dislocation in the adult. J Bone Joint Surg Am 1979;61(2):239–44.

Ulnar Collateral Ligament Injuries of the Thumb
A Comprehensive Review

Daniel M. Avery III, MD[a], Nicholas M. Caggiano, MD[a], Kristofer S. Matullo, MD[b],*

KEYWORDS

- Ulnar collateral ligament • Thumb • Metacarpophalangeal joint • Trauma

KEY POINTS

- Injuries to the thumb ulnar collateral ligament (UCL) are common. Failure to address the ensuing laxity of the metacarpophalangeal joint can lead to compromised grip and pinch, pain, and ultimately osteoarthritis.
- Patients who have sustained an acute injury commonly recount a traumatic episode with an accompanying onset of pain and swelling, whereas those with chronic injuries may present with less specific symptoms.
- The diagnosis of UCL injury relies primarily on the clinical examination of the patient.
- Instability to valgus stress with the lack of a firm end point is a strong indicator of complete rupture of the UCL. Ultrasonography, MRI, and plain films can be useful adjuncts.
- Nonoperative treatment is reserved for incomplete ruptures of the thumb UCL.
- Operative intervention is typically performed for complete ruptures.
- The goal of surgery is to restore the anatomic position of the ligament, thus providing stability to the metacarpophalangeal joint and allowing for protected range of motion early in the rehabilitation period.
- Both repair of acute ruptures and reconstruction for chronic injuries yield excellent results. Complications are rare and most patients show preservation of motion, key pinch, and grip strength.
- Range of motion exercises early in the rehabilitation phase help to ensure a positive outcome.

INTRODUCTION

Ulnar collateral ligament (UCL) injuries of the thumb are among the most common injuries in the hand.[1,2] In some populations, the incidence is as high as 50 per 100,000[3] and they are 10 times more common than their radial version.[4] Acute injuries, commonly referred to as skier's thumb,[5] have been known to occur in various sporting activities[6] in addition to their namesake, but are also common in manual laborers.[7] So-called gamekeeper's thumb, the chronic form of UCL insufficiency, has also been well documented.[8]

A stable, pain-free thumb base is not only essential for various sports and hobbies but also for activities of daily living, gripping, and key pinch. Insufficiency can lead to compromised grip and pinch, pain, and ultimately osteoarthritis. This article summarizes the current concepts in the management of these injuries in their acute and chronic forms.

The authors have nothing to disclose.
[a] Department of Orthopaedic Surgery, St. Luke's University Hospital, 801 Ostrum Street, PPH-2, Bethlehem, PA 18015, USA; [b] Division of Hand Surgery, Department of Orthopaedic Surgery, St. Luke's University Health Network, Bethlehem, PA 18015, USA
* Corresponding author.
E-mail address: kristofer.matullo@sluhn.org

orthopedic.theclinics.com

ANATOMY

The metacarpophalangeal joint (MCPJ) of the thumb is a diarthrodial ginglymoid (hinge) joint that has a variably flattened metacarpal head compared with its digital counterparts.[9] Its main range of motion is in flexion and extension with a lesser amount of abduction, adduction, and rotation.[10] The metacarpal head has a greater arc of curvature on the lateral condyle, which allows pronation with increasing flexion and enables opposition.[9]

Stability of the MCPJ is conferred by static and dynamic stabilizers, and to a lesser amount by the articular surface. The volar (or palmar) plate with its embedded 2 sesamoid bones and the radial collateral ligament and UCL provides static stabilization. Dynamic muscular stabilizers from the intrinsics include the abductor pollicis brevis (APB), flexor pollicis brevis, and adductor pollicis (AP), as well as stabilizers from the extrinsics with the extensor pollicis longus (EPL), extensor pollicis brevis (EPB), and flexor pollicis longus (FPL). The principal dynamic stabilizer is the AP, which resists valgus forces. The FPL and intrinsic musculature overpower the EPL and EPB, producing a primary volar pull on the proximal phalanx.[11]

The UCL is composed of 2 distinct structures or bundles: the proper UCL and accessory UCL.[10] The proper UCL originates from just below the metacarpal head and courses in a dorsal to palmar direction to insert on the base of the proximal phalanx.[12] The accessory UCL lies superficial and volar to the proper UCL, blending with the volar plate and inserting on the base of the proximal phalanx.[5] The primary function of the UCL is to provide resistance to valgus stress and volar subluxation.[13,14] In extension, the accessory UCL is tight, whereas the proper UCL is lax. At approximately 30° of flexion, the proper UCL is tight, whereas the accessory UCL slides proximally with the volar plate becoming lax (**Fig. 1**).[15] Normal valgus laxity is approximately 6° in extension and 12° in flexion.[16]

PATHOANATOMY

Injury to the UCL usually occurs as the result of hyperabduction or hyperextension of the MCPJ. This injury is commonly found among a high number of sports[6] and falls onto an outstretched hand.[11,17–20] The term skier's thumb was coined for its high incidence among skiers who fell, with the pole causing injury to the thumb.[5] Tearing of the UCL also commonly results in concomitant injury to the dorsal capsule and the volar plate leading to a volar subluxation of the proximal phalanx. This subluxation is caused by the palmar/radial force of the APB causing a radial shift.[9,21] Because the UCL travels dorsal to the flexion-extension axis, chronic UCL insufficiency can lead to a supination deformity at the proximal phalanx as it rotates around an intact radial collateral ligament.[14] Each of these deformities can be evident on clinical examination or radiographic assessment.

The UCL tear most commonly occurs at its distal insertion, sometimes as an avulsion fracture, but midstance and proximal ruptures do occur.[22–24] If the abduction force continues to pull the distal phalanx radially, the adductor aponeurosis can travel far enough distal to cause the UCL to lie superficial to the adductor aponeurosis. This condition is termed a Stener lesion and precludes the UCL from healing by nonoperative means.[22,25] This Stener lesion has been noted to occur in approximately 60% to 90% of cases, depending on the source.[22,26]

PHYSICAL EXAMINATION

After obtaining a thorough history, examination begins with inspection of the thumb. In acute injuries, swelling and ecchymosis are usually evident and volar radial subluxation may be visible with larger injuries. Pain is elicited on the ulnar aspect of the MCPJ with palpation. In some cases, a palpable mass may be evident, suggesting a Stener lesion.

Stress examination of the MCPJ is the most important evaluation of stability of the UCL[21] and should be compared with the contralateral side.[1] One hand should stabilize the metacarpal neck while the other grasps the proximal phalanx and controls rotation, because rotation of the phalanx

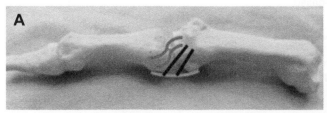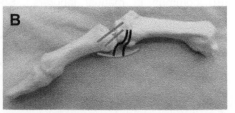

Fig. 1. UCLs (accessory and proper). The proper collateral ligament is shown at lax in extension (*A; wavy lines*) and tight in flexion (*B; straight lines*). The accessory ligament is tight in extension (*A*) and lax in flexion (*B*).

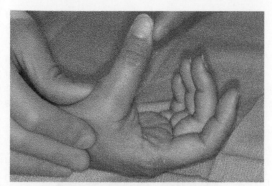

Fig. 2. Stress examination of the UCL. The examiner's right hand supports the metacarpal neck while exerting a valgus force with the left index finger.

can masquerade as valgus laxity (**Fig. 2**). Valgus stress should be applied to the thumb in full extension and in 30° of flexion.[15] Laxity of either 30° total or 15° more than the contralateral side suggests injury. If the laxity occurs in 30° of flexion alone, an injury to the proper UCL is suspected. If instability is noted in 30° of flexion and also in full extension, injury to the proper and accessory UCL is suspected.[27,28] If instability is noted only in extension, the volar plate may be the only injured structure.[29] Malik and colleagues[30] showed that a difference of 15° in flexion or extension can be normal in some patients, but the numbers stated earlier are traditionally accepted. Because of this variation, some clinicians prefer to place more emphasis on whether or not there is a firm end point to stress testing, which differentiates a partial from a complete injury.

Stressing the MCPJ in an acutely injured patient may be painful, with guarding or muscle spasm giving a false-negative examination. Local anesthesia can be injected into the MCPJ to allow for a better examination, which has been shown to increase accuracy from 28% to 98% in a study of 47 patients.[31]

DIAGNOSTIC STUDIES

Radiographs should always be obtained for patients with a history and physical examination suggesting a UCL tear. Radiographic assessment can identify avulsion fractures, isolated fractures of the proximal phalanx, or associated fractures of the metacarpal. Radial and volar subluxation can also be seen, as well as a supination deformity of the proximal phalanx relative to the metacarpal, termed the sag sign (**Fig. 3**).[32] Stress radiographs may be performed to better assess the degree of laxity in those patients with an equivocal clinical examination (**Fig. 4**). Some investigators suggest

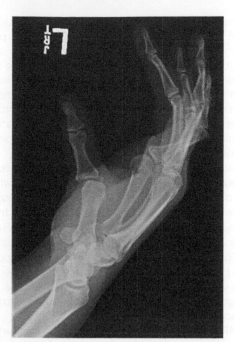

Fig. 3. Anteroposterior radiograph of the thumb showing the radial deviation and slight supination deformity at the MCPJ; the sag sign.

radiographic assessment before stressing the UCL because stress risks displacement of fracture fragments; however, if the initial energy was not strong enough to displace the fragment, then intra-office stress is not likely to be adequate to change

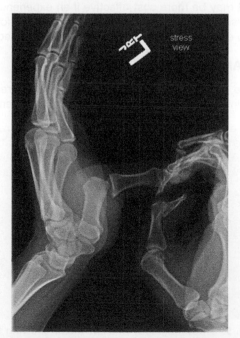

Fig. 4. Stress radiograph showing the gross valgus instability of the MCPJ that indicates a UCL injury.

its position.[33] Fractures, which can occur in up to 40% of injuries, are generally of 2 different patterns, as described by Hintermann and colleagues.[33] One is a true avulsion fracture and the other is an isolated fracture that is not associated with tear of the UCL. Differentiation can be made with stress radiographs. In a true avulsion fracture, stress in the radial direction causes further displacement of the fracture from the ulnar corner of the proximal phalanx.

Ultrasonography (US) is a noninvasive and cost-effective modality to evaluate for UCL tear when used along with clinical examination (**Fig. 5**). Results have varied widely, with accuracy ranging from 40% to 92%.[34,35] Review of the literature on US examination of UCL tears shows an overall sensitivity of 76%, specificity of 81%, accuracy of 81%, positive predictive value of 74%, and a negative predictive value of 87%.[36] Variability exists because the diagnostic value of US largely depends on the experience of the performing individual.

MRI is less cost-effective but more consistent in its ability to aid in the diagnosis of UCL tears, especially with dedicated extremity coils (**Fig. 6**). Arthrography has been shown to be even more accurate than MRI alone.[37,38] Hergan and colleagues[38] showed sensitivity and specificity of 100% with MRI versus 88% and 83% respectively with US.

It is the author's opinion that advanced imaging with US or MRI should be obtained in cases in which history or clinical examination is uncertain. US may be more cost-effective if an experienced musculoskeletal radiologist is available to perform the examination; if not, MRI should be obtained.

MANAGEMENT

The question of nonoperative or operative treatment is largely in debate but the decision depends

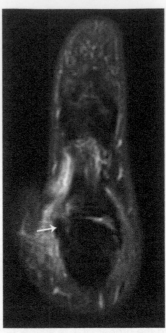

Fig. 6. T2 coronal MRI shows a tear of the UCL with the ligament retracted and confined proximally (*arrow*).

on stability and associated fractures. UCL injuries are generally categorized in grades. Grade I injuries, also termed sprains, are tender along the UCL but without increased laxity. Grade II injuries have increased laxity with a firm end point and are thought to be partial tears. Grade III injuries have both increased laxity and no firm end point, which indicates a complete tear. Grade I and II injuries are commonly treated nonoperatively.[14,39–41] Complete ruptures, with or without associated Stener lesions,[22,26] are treated surgically without consensus on optimal timing. Both repair and reconstruction have shown satisfactory results with regard to pain, strength, motion, and stability.[42] Unstable avulsion fractures are treated as grade III ligament injuries and isolated displaced fractures are treated with reduction and fixation of the articular segment.

NONOPERATIVE TREATMENT

Grade I and II injuries are appropriate for nonoperative treatment, because they are considered stable injuries. For these injuries with pain, mild laxity, and firm end points, immobilization is required to allow resolution of inflammation and to protect the MCPJ from further injury during the healing phase. The type of immobilization varies by clinician, but appropriate means include short-arm thumb spica casting, hand-based thumb spica

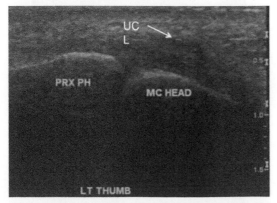

Fig. 5. Ultrasonography of a left thumb showing the metacarpal head (MC HEAD), proximal phalanx (PRX PH), and intact UCL.

casting, custom hand-based thermoplast splints, removable thumb spica splints, and functional hinged splints.[1,2,4,9,12,15,41] The important aspect is to protect the MCPJ from stress while allowing the interphalangeal (IP) joint of the thumb to move freely, thus avoiding undue stiffness.

Length of immobilization ranges from 10 days to 6 weeks depending on the extent of injury (sprain vs partial tear); however, immobilization for a period of 4 weeks is typically recommended.[1,2,6,9,12,15,27,29,41] Athletic participation is generally acceptable if the form of immobilization is permitted by local sporting regulations and use of the thumb is not required for that position or sport. At 4 weeks, occupational therapy or physiotherapy is initiated to regain motion, particularly in the flexion/extension plane, while avoiding valgus stresses at the MCPJ. At this time, immobilization is only required in high-risk activities, whether on the playing field or in the work or recreational environment. Strengthening begins at 6 to 8 weeks depending on the patient's progress, with unrestricted activity usually permitted at 12 weeks.

Nonoperative treatment has been reported in grade III injuries and UCL avulsion fractures with good results. Landsman and colleagues[43] and Pichora and colleagues[44] reported stable pain-free thumbs in 85% and 90% of their grade III injuries, respectively. However, the remaining patients in each study continued to have pain and instability, eventually requiring operative intervention. Pursuing nonoperative treatment of grade III injuries should be done cautiously and appropriate patient education should be performed at the outset.

Nonoperative treatment of UCL avulsion injuries has also shown mixed results in the literature. If there is a firm end point with a nondisplaced or minimally displaced fragment, immobilization alone can be considered. Kuz and colleagues[45] and Sorene and Goodwin[46] showed that, despite a 20% and 60% fibrous union rate respectively, all their nonoperatively treated patients were satisfied with their outcomes. This finding is in contrast with reports by Dinowitz and colleagues[47] and Bowers and Hurst[39] who reported persistent pain and instability after immobilization in all or nearly all of their patients, with most requiring eventual operative treatment. Dinowitz and colleagues[47] showed that triangular-shaped articular avulsion fragments may undergo rotation whereby the articular surface rotates into the fracture gap, whereas plain radiographs often appear to show a simple nondisplaced fracture. Close scrutiny is required to avoid mischaracterization of these seemingly nondisplaced fractures that are certain to lead to nonunion and likely posttraumatic arthritis, pain, and stiffness.

OPERATIVE TREATMENT

Indications for surgical exploration of the thumb UCL include grade III injuries, defined as greater than 30° of valgus deviation, 15° more laxity compared with the contralateral side, or lack of a firm end point.[48] Diagnostic imaging is used in equivocal cases of UCL injury. The goal of both surgical repair and reconstruction of the UCL is to reproduce the anatomic position of the ligament, restore stability to the MCPJ, and allow protected range of motion early in the rehabilitation period.

ACUTE ULNAR COLLATERAL LIGAMENT REPAIR

Acute, complete ruptures less than 3 to 6 weeks old are generally treated with repair of the anatomic ligament.[49] Acute ligament repair requires the native tissue to be of adequate length and quality. If the tissue is lacking in either length or quality, reconstruction should be undertaken in lieu of an inadequate repair.[50] As such, both the surgeon and patient must be prepared for the possibility that a reconstruction may need to be performed.

A variety of procedures exist for acute repair of the UCL. Although midsubstance tears are less common than distal tears, they can be treated with direct suture repair with a 3-0 or 4-0 nonabsorbable suture (**Fig. 7**).[51] Surgeons have the option of immobilizing the MCPJ with a K-wire for 4 weeks to protect the MCPJ from stress during the healing phase.[49]

Ligament disruptions occurring proximally at the metacarpal origin or, more commonly, at the insertion on the proximal phalanx are treated with surgical reattachment of the ligament to the bone. Options include transosseous pullout sutures through bone tunnels and suture anchors. Regardless of the method used, recreation of the anatomic footprint of the ligament is essential, because nonanatomic repositioning of the UCL leads to abnormal motion at the MCPJ,[52] which can predispose to posttraumatic arthritis or increased stiffness.

The approach to the MCPJ is performed via a lazy-S incision on the dorsal-ulnar aspect of the thumb (**Fig. 8**). This incision is performed to address any tear location because the metacarpal origin of the UCL is more dorsal and fans to a more distal and volar insertion on the proximal phalanx. Meticulous dissection is performed with the assistance of electrocautery to reach the adductor aponeurosis. Branches of the superficial radial nerve of the thumb, providing dorsal sensation, cross through the subcutaneous layer and should be identified and preserved.

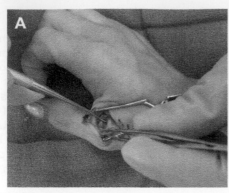 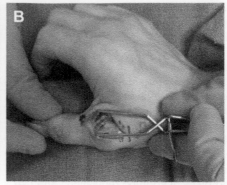

Fig. 7. (*A*) Demonstration of a midsubstance tear of the UCL. (*B*) Repair of a midsubstance tear of the UCL via transligamentous 4-0 sutures.

Once the adductor aponeurosis is exposed, the surgeon should attempt to locate the proximal limb of the torn UCL. A Stener lesion appears as a mass of tissue lying on the proximal border of the aponeurosis. A longitudinal incision is made in the adductor aponeurosis, favoring a slightly volar direction to expose the capsular surfaces of the MCPJ as well as the volar plate. The joint capsule is then split longitudinally at the dorsal border of the ligament (**Fig. 9**). At this point the MCPJ is examined. Any large fractures amenable to fixation are secured anatomically, whereas any small bony or cartilaginous avulsion fragments that are deemed too small for repair are excised.

The bony site of injury should be debrided to bleeding bone to encourage ligament-to-bone healing (**Fig. 10**). On the metacarpal, the origin of the ligament is 7 mm proximal to the joint surface, 3 mm from the dorsal border, and 8 mm from the volar surface.[52] The site of insertion on the proximal phalanx is 3 mm distal to the joint surface, 8 mm from the dorsal border, and 3 mm from the volar surface.[52]

When performing a suture pullout technique, the end of the ligament stump should be cleaned with a 15 blade to remove any loose remnants. A 3-0 nonabsorbable suture is secured to the ligament stump by means of a Kessler or Bunnell stitch. At the proximal phalanx (for distal ruptures) or the metacarpal (for proximal ruptures), 2 drill holes are created transversely, both starting on the ulnar site of ligament attachment. The holes should be drilled to exit on the dorsoradial aspect of the thumb and be slightly divergent to maximize the bony bridge on the far radial cortex.[53] Fluoroscopy is useful to ensure the accuracy of the bone tunnel position. The suture ends are then passed through the bone tunnels with a Keith needle. The thumb is held with the MCPJ in 15° of flexion and slight ulnar deviation. The suture is appropriately tensioned and the ends are either tied outside the skin over a button or tied directly over the bony bridge under the skin.

The suture anchor technique uses a similar exposure and debridement of bony landmarks to encourage ligament-to-bone healing. A small suture anchor is placed at the site of origin on the metacarpal or at the site of insertion on the proximal phalanx. Again, fluoroscopy is useful to ensure accurate positioning of the anchor and to verify extra-articular placement of the anchor. The thumb

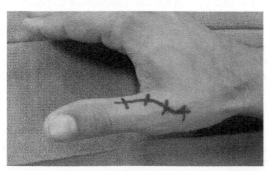 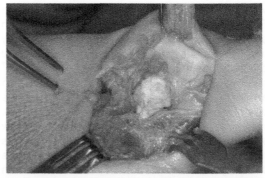

Fig. 8. Lazy-S incision drawn over the dorsal-ulnar aspect of the MCPJ.

Fig. 9. Meticulous surgical dissection readily shows the adductor aponeurosis and torn UCL.

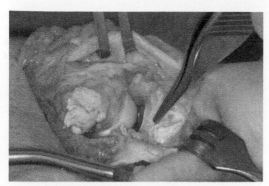

Fig. 10. Deep dissection reveals the torn UCL attached to the proximal metacarpal head and the insertion site at the base of the proximal phalanx (tip forceps).

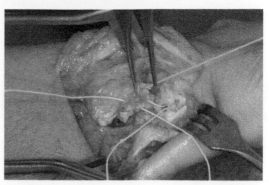

Fig. 12. Double-loaded suture is passed through the torn ligament.

is then held with the MCPJ in 15° of flexion and slight ulnar deviation. The sutures are tensioned and secured to the ligament stump with a Kessler or Bunnell stitch pulling the ligament to lie in contact with the prepared bony area (**Figs. 11–13**).

Regardless of the type of repair used, the accessory portion of the UCL should be assessed following repair of the proper ligament. If preoperative examination reveals laxity to ulnar stress in extension, the accessory portion is most likely violated. In such a case, a 3-0 nonabsorbable suture is used to repair the accessory portion to the ulnar aspect of the volar plate.[49]

After the ligament has been repaired, the wound is copiously irrigated. Both the joint capsule and the adductor aponeurosis are closed with a 4-0 absorbable suture.[50] The skin is closed according to surgeon preference and a forearm-based thumb spica splint is applied with preservation of motion at the IP joint of the thumb.

Although both the pullout suture technique and suture anchor technique have shown successful patient outcomes,[14,42,53] recent studies have shown that suture anchor fixation results in improved pinch strength, better motion, reduced

operating time, and fewer complications.[2,5,51,53–55] The pullout suture technique is technically more demanding compared with suture anchor fixation.[53] Suture anchors provide predictable and reliable fixation with the ability to allow active range of motion early in the rehabilitation period.[55,56] Complications are few and include failure of primary repair, infection, paresthesias on the radial border of the thumb, and decreased range of motion.[2,14,23,53,57]

CHRONIC ULNAR COLLATERAL LIGAMENT RECONSTRUCTION

Injuries greater than 3 weeks old have historically had poor outcomes with surgical repair, presumably because of attenuation of the remnant ligament.[1,14,21,26] Reconstruction is a better option for these older injuries if the tissue quality or length is inappropriate for primary repair. Even in the setting of well-documented acute injury, a careful and thorough history is necessary because preinjury thumb pain or instability may indicate an acute on chronic injury. Furthermore, plain films should be obtained and examined for evidence of arthritis,

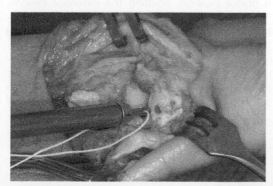

Fig. 11. Suture anchor placement in the center of the anatomic footprint.

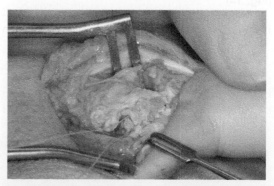

Fig. 13. The ligament is then reapproximated to its distal insertion on the proximal phalanx.

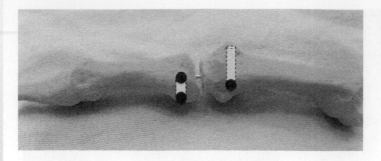

Fig. 14. Drill tunnels for UCL reconstruction. Two converging holes in the proximal phalanx on the ulnar side and 1 tunnel across the metacarpal head from ulnar to radial.

because this is a contraindication to UCL reconstruction.

The palmaris longus tendon, if present, is typically used for tendon graft reconstruction of the UCL.[14,49] Some investigators have described using a slip of the abductor pollicis longus,[58] mobilizing the proximal aspect of the EPB tendon,[25] or harvesting the fourth toe extensor for use as graft.[59] Similar variation exists with regard to the configuration of bone tunnels. Both apex-proximal[60] and apex-distal[61] triangular patterns have been described, along with figure-of-eight[59] and rectangular patterns.[28] For the sake of brevity, only the use of a palmaris longus graft inserted in an apex-proximal configuration is discussed here.

After harvest of the palmaris longus graft, exposure of the MCPJ is performed as described earlier. A valgus stress should be applied to the MCPJ to thoroughly examine the articular surfaces. Once the surgeon is convinced that the joint is not arthritic, 2 bone tunnels are created in the proximal phalanx at the 1 and 4 o'clock (left thumb) or 11 and 8 o'clock positions (right thumb) when viewing the digit end on.[60] The tunnels are centered over the anatomic footprint of the UCL ulnarly and are drilled at 45° angles radially. The tunnels converge in the intramedullary cavity. A single metacarpal tunnel is created transversely from ulnar to radial at the anatomic origin of the UCL (**Fig. 14**).

The graft is passed through the phalangeal tunnels. The ends of the graft are then passed through the metacarpal from ulnar to radial using a 28-gauge stainless steel wire or a suture passer (**Fig. 15**). The thumb is held with the MCPJ at 15° of flexion and slight ulnar deviation. The graft is then secured in the metacarpal with either an interference screw or the graft ends are tied in a knot and sutured to the periosteum on the radial aspect of the thumb. The wound is irrigated and closed as described earlier, and a forearm-based splint is placed to immobilize the MCPJ while preserving motion at the thumb IP joint.

Despite the variety of options available for reconstruction of the chronically injured thumb UCL, outcomes are consistently good to excellent.[60,62,63] Patients show up to 91% of key pinch and grip strength[60,62] and 90% stability compared with the uninjured side.[60] Complications include pain, infection, loss of range of motion,[14] and (rarely) hyperextension laxity.[28] Reconstruction remains a viable alternative treatment of UCL injuries not amenable to primary repair.

THE ARTHRITIC JOINT

Thumb MCPJ instability in the setting of osteoarthritis is best served with a joint arthrodesis. Restabilization via reconstruction tends to reconstrain the joint and may result in increased pain in the postoperative period. Exposure is via a dorsal incision, splitting the extensor interval. The joint surfaces are denuded of articular cartilage to bleeding subchondral bone and

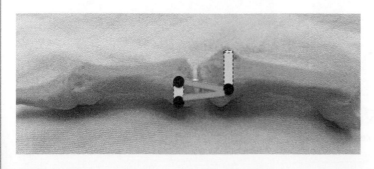

Fig. 15. Graft is passed through the proximal phalanx and then both limbs are passed from ulnar to radial through the metacarpal head.

arthrodesis is accomplished via cannulated screws,[64] K-wire and tension band fixation (**Fig. 16**),[65] or a plate and screw construct (**Fig. 17**). The MCPJ should be immobilized for 4 to 6 weeks or until there is radiographic evidence of fusion. Excellent results can be expected, with fusion rates nearing 100%.[66] Patients usually find an increase in key pinch strength compared with preoperative testing, but may complain of mild postoperative pain or difficulty with picking up small objects. Overall, success rates are high with arthrodesis for the arthritic MCPJ.[64,66]

POSTOPERATIVE MANAGEMENT

The MCPJ of the thumb is immobilized postoperatively in a forearm-based thumb spica splint. The IP joint is left free to prevent adhesions of the EPL tendon. Recent evidence has shown that early active range of motion is safe following suture anchor fixation.[56,67] In this protocol, the forearm-based thumb spica splint is removed at postoperative day 3 to 5 and is replaced by a removable thermoplastic splint. Patients are instructed to come out of the splint 4 times per day for active range of motion exercises. The splint is discontinued at week 4 for general activities with continued therapy for strengthening and range of motion exercises. The splint is used for sports or other stressful activities involving the MCPJ. Full return to activities is allowed at 3 months.[68]

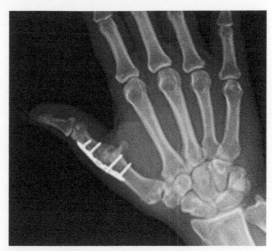

Fig. 17. Arthrodesis of the thumb MCPJ using a plate and screw construct.

SUMMARY

Injuries to the thumb UCL are common. Failure to address the ensuing laxity of the MCPJ can lead to compromised grip and pinch, pain, and ultimately osteoarthritis. Patients who have sustained an acute injury commonly recount a traumatic episode with an accompanying onset of pain and swelling, whereas those with chronic injuries may present with less specific symptoms.

The diagnosis of UCL injury relies primarily on the clinical examination of the patient. Instability to valgus stress with the lack of a firm end point is a strong indicator of complete rupture of the UCL. Ultrasonography, MRI, and plain films can be useful adjuncts.

Nonoperative treatment is reserved for incomplete ruptures of the thumb UCL. Operative intervention is typically performed for complete ruptures. The goal of surgery is to restore the anatomic position of the ligament, thus providing stability to the MCPJ and allowing protected range of motion early in the rehabilitation period.

Both repair of acute ruptures and reconstruction for chronic injuries yield excellent results. Complications are rare and most patients show preservation of motion, key pinch, and grip strength. Range of motion exercises early in the rehabilitation phase help to ensure a positive outcome.

REFERENCES

1. Rhee PC, Jones DB, Kakar S. Management of thumb metacarpophalangeal ulnar collateral ligament injuries. J Bone Joint Surg Am 2012;94(21):2005–12.
2. Baskies MA, Lee SK. Evaluation and treatment of injuries of the ulnar collateral ligament of the thumb

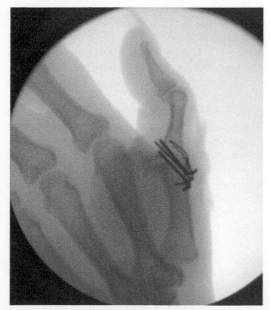

Fig. 16. Arthrodesis of the thumb MCPJ using K-wires and a tension band construct.

metacarpophalangeal joint. Bull NYU Hosp Jt Dis 2009;67(1):68–74.

3. Jones MH, England SJ, Muwanga CL, et al. The use of ultrasound in the diagnosis of injuries of the ulnar collateral ligament of the thumb. J Hand Surg Br 2000;25(1):29–32.

4. Keramidas E, Miller G. Adult hand injuries on artificial ski slopes. Ann Plast Surg 2005;55(4):357–8.

5. Gerber C, Senn E, Matter P. Skier's thumb. Surgical treatment of recent injuries to the ulnar collateral ligament of the thumb's metacarpophalangeal joint. Am J Sports Med 1981;9(3):171–7.

6. Lee AT, Carlson MG. Thumb metacarpophalangeal joint collateral ligament injury management. Hand Clin 2012;28(3):361–70, ix–x.

7. Chuter GS, Muwanga CL, Irwin LR. Ulnar collateral ligament injuries of the thumb: 10 years of surgical experience. Injury 2009;40(6):652–6.

8. Campbell CS. Gamekeeper's thumb. J Bone Joint Surg Br 1955;37-B(1):148–9.

9. Johnson JW, Culp RW. Acute ulnar collateral ligament injury in the athlete. Hand Clin 2009;25(3):437–42.

10. Frank WE, Dobyns J. Surgical pathology of collateral ligamentous injuries of the thumb. Clin Orthop Relat Res 1972;83:102–14.

11. Posner MA, Retaillaud JL. Metacarpophalangeal joint injuries of the thumb. Hand Clin 1992;8(4):713–32.

12. Stener B. Hyperextension injuries to the metacarpophalangeal joint of the thumb: rupture of ligaments, fracture of sesamoid bones, rupture of flexor pollicis brevis. An anatomical and clinical study. Acta Chir Scand 1963;125:275–93.

13. Cooney WP 3rd, Chao EY. Biomechanical analysis of static forces in the thumb during hand function. J Bone Joint Surg Am 1977;59(1):27–36.

14. Smith RJ. Post-traumatic instability of the metacarpophalangeal joint of the thumb. J Bone Joint Surg Am 1977;59(1):14–21.

15. Moberg E, Stener B. Injuries to the ligaments of the thumb and fingers; diagnosis, treatment and prognosis. Acta Chir Scand 1953;106(2–3):166–86.

16. Coonrad RW, Goldner JL. A study of the pathological findings and treatment in soft-tissue injury of the thumb metacarpophalangeal joint. With a clinical study of the normal range of motion in one thousand thumbs and a study of post mortem findings of ligamentous structures in relation to function. J Bone Joint Surg Am 1968;50(3):439–51.

17. Bailie DS, Benson LS, Marymont JV. Proximal interphalangeal joint injuries of the hand. Part I: anatomy and diagnosis. Am J Orthop (Belle Mead NJ) 1996;25(7):474–7.

18. Benson LS, Bailie DS. Proximal interphalangeal joint injuries of the hand. Part II: treatment and complications. Am J Orthop (Belle Mead NJ) 1996;25(8):527–30.

19. Melone CP Jr, Beldner S, Basuk RS. Thumb collateral ligament injuries. An anatomic basis for treatment. Hand Clin 2000;16(3):345–57.

20. Van Dommelen BA, Zvirbulis RA. Upper extremity injuries in snow skiers. Am J Sports Med 1989;17(6):751–3.

21. Tang P. Collateral ligament injuries of the thumb metacarpophalangeal joint. J Am Acad Orthop Surg 2011;19(5):287–96.

22. Stener B. Displacement of the ruptured ulnar collateral ligament of the metacarpophalangeal joint of the thumb. J Bone Joint Surg Br 1962;44-B:869–79.

23. Derkash RS, et al. Acute surgical repair of the skier's thumb. Clin Orthop Relat Res 1987;(216):29–33.

24. Palmer AK, Louis DS. Assessing ulnar instability of the metacarpophalangeal joint of the thumb. J Hand Surg Am 1978;3(6):542–6.

25. Strandell G. Total rupture of the ulnar collateral ligament of the metacarpophalangeal joint of the thumb: results of surgery in 35 cases. Acta Chir Scand 1959;118:72–80.

26. Heyman P, et al. Injuries of the ulnar collateral ligament of the thumb metacarpophalangeal joint. Biomechanical and prospective clinical studies on the usefulness of valgus stress testing. Clin Orthop Relat Res 1993;(292):165–71.

27. Morgan WJ, Slowman LS. Acute hand and wrist injuries in athletes: evaluation and management. J Am Acad Orthop Surg 2001;9(6):389–400.

28. Osterman AL, Hayken GD, Bora FW Jr. A quantitative evaluation of thumb function after ulnar collateral repair and reconstruction. J Trauma 1981;21(10):854–61.

29. Lee SJ, Montgomery K. Athletic hand injuries. Orthop Clin North Am 2002;33(3):547–54.

30. Malik AK, et al. Clinical testing of ulnar collateral ligament injuries of the thumb. J Hand Surg Eur Vol 2009;34(3):363–6.

31. Cooper JG, et al. Local anaesthetic infiltration increases the accuracy of assessment of ulnar collateral ligament injuries. Emerg Med Australas 2005;17(2):132–6.

32. Gurdezi S, Mok D. 'Sag Sign' - A simple radiological sign for detecting injury to the thumb ulnar collateral ligament. Injury Extra 2008;39(5):155–208.

33. Hintermann B, et al. Skier's thumb–the significance of bony injuries. Am J Sports Med 1993;21(6):800–4.

34. Hergan K, Mittler C. Sonography of the injured ulnar collateral ligament of the thumb. J Bone Joint Surg Br 1995;77(1):77–83.

35. Susic D, Hansen BR, Hansen TB. Ultrasonography may be misleading in the diagnosis of ruptured and dislocated ulnar collateral ligaments of the thumb. Scand J Plast Reconstr Surg Hand Surg 1999;33(3):319–20.

36. Papandrea RF, Fowler T. Injury at the thumb UCL: is there a Stener lesion? J Hand Surg Am 2008;33(10):1882–4.

37. Ahn JM, et al. Gamekeeper thumb: comparison of MR arthrography with conventional arthrography and MR imaging in cadavers. Radiology 1998; 206(3):737–44.

38. Hergan K, Mittler C, Oser W. Ulnar collateral ligament: differentiation of displaced and nondisplaced tears with US and MR imaging. Radiology 1995; 194(1):65–71.

39. Bowers WH, Hurst LC. Gamekeeper's thumb. Evaluation by arthrography and stress roentgenography. J Bone Joint Surg Am 1977;59(4):519–24.

40. Abrahamsson SO, et al. Diagnosis of displaced ulnar collateral ligament of the metacarpophalangeal joint of the thumb. J Hand Surg Am 1990;15(3): 457–60.

41. Sollerman C, et al. Functional splinting versus plaster cast for ruptures of the ulnar collateral ligament of the thumb. A prospective randomized study of 63 cases. Acta Orthop Scand 1991;62(6):524–6.

42. Samora JB, et al. Outcomes after injury to the thumb ulnar collateral ligament–a systematic review. Clin J Sport Med 2013;23(4):247–54.

43. Landsman JC, et al. Splint immobilization of gamekeeper's thumb. Orthopedics 1995;18(12): 1161–5.

44. Pichora DR, McMurtry RY, Bell MJ. Gamekeepers thumb: a prospective study of functional bracing. J Hand Surg Am 1989;14(3):567–73.

45. Kuz JE, et al. Outcome of avulsion fractures of the ulnar base of the proximal phalanx of the thumb treated nonsurgically. J Hand Surg Am 1999;24(2): 275–82.

46. Sorene ED, Goodwin DR. Non-operative treatment of displaced avulsion fractures of the ulnar base of the proximal phalanx of the thumb. Scand J Plast Reconstr Surg Hand Surg 2003;37(4):225–7.

47. Dinowitz M, et al. Failure of cast immobilization for thumb ulnar collateral ligament avulsion fractures. J Hand Surg Am 1997;22(6):1057–63.

48. Ritting AW, Baldwin PC, Rodner CM. Ulnar collateral ligament injury of the thumb metacarpophalangeal joint. Clin J Sport Med 2010;20(2):106–12.

49. Badia A, Prakash K. Arthroscopic and open primary repair of acute thumb metacarpophalangeal joint radial and ulnar collateral ligament disruptions. In: Wiesel SW, editor. Operative techniques in orthopaedic surgery. Philadelphia: Lippincott Williams & Wilkins; 2010. p. 2342–8.

50. Merrell G, Joseph F. Dislocations and ligament injuries in the digits. In: Green DP, Wolfe SW, editors. Green's operative hand surgery. Philadelphia: Elsevier/ Churchill Livingstone; 2011. p. 291–332.

51. Tsiouri C, Hayton MJ, Baratz M. Injury to the ulnar collateral ligament of the thumb. Hand (N Y) 2009; 4(1):12–8.

52. Bean CH, Tencer AF, Trumble TE. The effect of thumb metacarpophalangeal ulnar collateral ligament attachment site on joint range of motion: an in vitro study. J Hand Surg Am 1999;24(2): 283–7.

53. Katolik LI, Friedrich J, Trumble TE. Repair of acute ulnar collateral ligament injuries of the thumb metacarpophalangeal joint: a retrospective comparison of pull-out sutures and bone anchor techniques. Plast Reconstr Surg 2008;122(5): 1451–6.

54. Zeman C, et al. Acute skier's thumb repaired with a proximal phalanx suture anchor. Am J Sports Med 1998;26(5):644–50.

55. Moharram AN. Repair of thumb metacarpophalangeal joint ulnar collateral ligament injuries with microanchors. Ann Plast Surg 2013;71(5): 500–2.

56. Crowley TP, et al. Early active mobilization following UCL repair with Mitek bone anchor. Tech Hand Up Extrem Surg 2013;17(3):124–7.

57. Weiland AJ, et al. Repair of acute ulnar collateral ligament injuries of the thumb metacarpophalangeal joint with an intraosseous suture anchor. J Hand Surg Am 1997;22(4):585–91.

58. Frykman G, Johansson O. Surgical repair of rupture of the ulnar collateral ligament of the metacarpophalangeal joint of the thumb. Acta Chir Scand 1956;112(1):58–64.

59. Alldred AJ. Rupture of the collateral ligament of the metacarpo-phalangeal joint of the thumb. J Bone Joint Surg Br 1955;37-B(3):443–5.

60. Glickel SZ, et al. Ligament replacement for chronic instability of the ulnar collateral ligament of the metacarpophalangeal joint of the thumb. J Hand Surg Am 1993;18(5):930–41.

61. Fairhurst M, Hansen L. Treatment of "Gamekeeper's Thumb" by reconstruction of the ulnar collateral ligament. J Hand Surg Br 2002;27(6):542–5.

62. Oka Y, Harayama H, Ikeda M. Reconstructive procedure to repair chronic injuries to the collateral ligament of metacarpophalangeal joints of the hand. Hand Surg 2003;8(1):81–5.

63. Wong TC, Ip FK, Wu WC. Bone-periosteum-bone graft reconstruction for chronic ulnar instability of the metacarpophalangeal joint of the thumb–minimum 5-year follow-up evaluation. J Hand Surg Am 2009;34(2):304–8.

64. Schmidt CC, Zimmer SM, Boles SD. Arthrodesis of the thumb metacarpophalangeal joint using a cannulated screw and threaded washer. J Hand Surg Am 2004;29(6):1044–50.

65. Rizzo M. Metacarpophalangeal joint arthritis. J Hand Surg Am 2011;36(2):345–53.

66. Hagan HJ, Hastings H 2nd. Fusion of the thumb metacarpophalangeal joint to treat posttraumatic arthritis. J Hand Surg Am 1988;13(5):750–3.

67. Harley BJ, Werner FW, Green JK. A biomechanical modeling of injury, repair, and rehabilitation of ulnar

collateral ligament injuries of the thumb. J Hand Surg Am 2004;29(5):915–20.

68. Little KJ, Sidney JM. Intra-articular hand fractures and joint injuries: Part I - surgeon's management.

In: Skirven TM, editor. Rehabilitation of the hand and upper extremity. Philadelphia: Elsevier Mosby; 2011. p. 1. online resource (2 v. (xxxv, 1889, I-61 p.)).

Evaluation and Nonsurgical Management of Rotator Cuff Calcific Tendinopathy

Ari C. Greis, DO[a],*, Stephen M. Derrington, DO[b], Matthew McAuliffe, MD[b]

KEYWORDS

- Rotator cuff • Calcific tendinopathy • Shoulder pain • Ultrasound • Aspiration • Lavage

KEY POINTS

- Rotator cuff calcific tendinopathy is a common asymptomatic finding on imaging studies that accounts for shoulder pain in approximately 7% of cases.
- Most patients can be managed conservatively with a combination of nonsteroidal anti-inflammatory drugs, modalities, physical therapy, and injection therapy.
- The goal of physical therapy is to improve scapular mechanics and decrease subacromial impingement.
- Ultrasound-guided needle aspiration and lavage of calcium deposits in the rotator cuff tendons have been shown to decrease the size of deposits and improve pain and function on a long-term basis.

INTRODUCTION

Rotator cuff disease is a common cause of shoulder pain. The differential diagnosis of rotator cuff disease includes tendinitis, tendinopathy, subacromial Impingement, partial and full thickness tendon tears, and calcific tendinopathy. Although calcific tendinopathy is a common incidental finding on imaging studies, it can also be a cause of significant shoulder pain and disability. The supraspinatus tendon is most commonly involved, which can lead to significant subacromial impingement and limit activities at or above shoulder level. Like many other rotator cuff problems, most patients respond well to relative rest, nonsteroidal anti-inflammatory drugs (NSAIDs), physical therapy, and subacromial bursa injections with corticosteroids. There is growing interest and use of ultrasound-guided injection procedures in musculoskeletal medicine. One novel technique for the treatment of rotator cuff calcific tendinopathy (RCCT) involves advancing a larger-gauge needle under live sonography into the calcium deposit, fragmenting it, and aspirating its contents. This technique has been shown to provide excellent long-term pain relief and may be a good alternative to surgical intervention.

EPIDEMIOLOGY

There have been several studies on the epidemiology of RCCT. One of the most famous of these

The authors have nothing to disclose.
[a] Department of Physical Medicine and Rehabilitation, Rothman Institute, Thomas Jefferson University, 925 Chestnut Street, Philadelphia, PA 19107, USA; [b] Department of Physical Medicine and Rehabilitation, Thomas Jefferson University, 25 South 9th Street, Philadelphia, PA 19107, USA
* Corresponding author. Rothman Institute, 170 North Henderson Road, King of Prussia, PA 19406.
E-mail address: arigreis@gmail.com

Orthop Clin N Am 46 (2015) 293–302
http://dx.doi.org/10.1016/j.ocl.2014.11.011
0030-5898/15/$ – see front matter © 2015 Elsevier Inc. All rights reserved.

studies was done in 1941 by Bosworth,[1] who looked at 5061 office employees and found the prevalence of calcium deposits in the rotator cuff to be 2.7% on fluoroscopic examination. Several other studies have reported prevalence rates ranging from 2.7% to 22%, mostly affecting people ranging from 30 to 50 years of age.[1–3] It is often an asymptomatic finding on imaging studies. However, when considering people with shoulder pain, RCCT is a finding 6.8% of the time.[4] When one shoulder is affected, the other shoulder will also be affected 14% of the time.[5] Similar to other rotator cuff pathologic abnormalities, the supraspinatus tendon is most likely to be affected.[3]

People with sedentary lifestyles experience a higher risk of developing RCCT.[4] Ischemic heart disease, hypertension, diabetes, and thyroid disease are known associated medical conditions that seem to predispose patients to developing calcific tendinopathy for reasons not well understood.[6] There is a known correlation with calcific tendinopathy and endocrine disorders. These patients have an earlier onset of symptoms, a longer disease course, and ultimately undergo surgery more frequently than people that do not have these conditions.[7] Interestingly, RCCT is rarely associated with metabolic disorders related to calcium or phosphorus.[5]

PATHOPHYSIOLOGY

The mechanism of the pathogenesis of calcific tendinopathy has remained elusive. There are several competing theories. It has been suggested that one of the reasons the pathogenesis remains unknown is that biopsies obtained are done near the end of the natural history of the disease.[8,9] The other theories on the pathogenesis of calcific tendinopathy that will be discussed in this article include degenerative calcification, reactive calcification, endochondral ossification, and chondral metaplasia (**Table 1**).

In degenerative calcification, it has been proposed that tendon fibers deteriorate over time. It is thought that aging tenocytes become progressively more damaged with time as a result of decreased vascular flow and tendon fibers become hypocellular and eventually undergo necrosis from the damage.[3,10–12] As a result, intracellular calcium builds within the tenocytes in the form of psammoma bodies during the beginning phases of calcification; this in turn becomes larger over time until there are macroscopic areas of calcification that will be apparent on imaging and possibly symptomatic in affected patients.[3,8,12]

Reactive calcification proposes the cause of calcification as a multistage process beginning

Table 1
Summary of different theories on pathogenesis of calcific tendinopathy

Theory	Proposed Mechanism
Degenerative calcification	Intracellular calcium accumulated from old, damaged, and necrotic tenocytes
Reactive calcification	Metaplastic fibrocartilage with calcium deposited through an inflammatory mechanism
Endochondral ossification	Metaplastic fibrocartilage becomes vascular from underlying bone marrow and calcium deposited without evidence of inflammation (similar to bone spur formation)
Chondral metaplasia	Erroneous differentiation of tenocytes into bone cells, mediated by BMP-2

with tenocyte metaplasia, which leads to calcification and ultimately a cell-mediated inflammatory reaction.[9] Uhthoff and colleagues[9] proposed dividing the process into 3 main stages: precalcific, calcific, and postcalcific (**Table 2**). In the precalcific stage, the tenocytes undergo metaplasia into fibrocartilaginous tissue, acting as a substrate for calcium deposition, which is thought to be mediated by chondrocytes.[3,9] The calcific stage is when actual calcium deposition occurs in the tendon and the body's subsequent reaction to a calcified tendon. Uhthoff and Loehr[3] further subdivide the calcific stage into the formative and resorptive phases. In the formative phase, calcium crystals deposit into the affected tissue, which is mediated by the chondrocytes of the metaplastic

Table 2
Summary of different stages of calcific tendinopathy

Stages of Calcification	Pathophysiology
Precalcific stage	Tenocytes undergo metaplasia into fibrocartilagenous tissue
Calcific stage: formative phase	Calcium crystals deposit onto metaplastic tissue
Calcific stage: resorptive phase	Phagocytosis of deposited calcium
Postcalcific stage	Remodeling of affected tissue

fibrocartilagenous tissue, that eventually combine into larger areas of calcified tissue. Uhthoff further comments that if surgery is done during this stage of the disease, the calcified areas will be chalky and need to be "scooped" out. The resorptive phase begins after a varying period of dormancy in the disease course. The affected area develops "vascular channels" wherein macrophages phagocytose and eliminate the calcium.[3,9] Finally, the postcalcific phase describes the process whereby fibroblasts in granulation tissue remodel the affected tissue following calcium removal.[3,9]

Another mechanism proposed by Benjamin and colleagues,[13] who studied Achilles tendons of rats, suggested that endochondral ossification of fibrocartilage is the pathogenesis of calcific tendinopathy.[8] Again, fibrocartilage first develops in affected sites through the process of metaplasia. The fibrocartilage then develops vascular flow from underlying bone marrow. As the fibrocartilage becomes increasingly vascular, deposits of calcium form.[13] What develops is essentially a bone spur in the tendon tissue.[8,13] An important note, through this process no inflammatory reaction was seen to take place.[13] Unfortunately, Benjamin and colleagues did not report on the process of resorption and changes that take place in the rat tendons.

The fourth mechanism discussed here is that of chondral metaplasia. Rui and colleagues[14] think the calcification of tenocytes is a result of erroneous differentiation of tendon stem cells into bone cells. Hashimoto and colleagues[15] showed that injection of bone morphogenic protein (BMP-2) into tendons produced ectopic bone formation in the tendon, suggesting tendon stem cells were responsive to proteins thought to induce bone growth. The exact mechanism by which tendon stem cells differentiate themselves incorrectly into bone is not clear at this point.

To complement the discussion, it has been proposed that there are genetic components that predispose certain populations to developing calcific tendinopathy.[6] It should also be mentioned again that there are several endocrine and vascular disorders that are associated with calcific tendinopathy. However, it is not clear how they affect the natural history of the disease.

Although the exact mechanism of the pathophysiology remains elusive, there are a few important points to take into consideration:

- There are several things that likely contribute to the development of calcific tendinopathy.
- There are several medical conditions that can predispose a person to this condition.
- There may be a genetic component and familial predisposition.

It is tempting to think there is some sort of injury that first occurs to the tendon cells, whether it is an acute clinically apparent injury or a series of subclinical microtraumas over the span of several years. Certainly, something must occur to induce metaplasia of the tenocytes that ultimately lead to the development of calcific tendinopathy. Furthermore, it is unclear if the calcification and resorption process are a part of normal healing that takes place in an injured tendon.

CLINICAL PRESENTATION

Calcific tendinopathy of the shoulder may present in several different ways; however, the main complaint when patients are symptomatic is pain. As previously discussed, epidemiologic studies have shown that many cases of calcific tendinopathy of the shoulder will be asymptomatic or an incidental finding on imaging studies. However, Bosworth[1] reported that 34% to 45% of patients with rotator cuff calcifications were found to be symptomatic.

A good way to look at RCCT, and its typical natural history, is that the disease progresses through 3 stages: the precalcification stage; the calcification stage, which includes the formative and resorptive phases; and the postcalcific stage (see **Table 2**).

Often, the pain is worse in acute presentations than in chronic presentations.[2,5] In some chronic forms, there may be periods whereby patients are asymptomatic and a relapsing remitting pattern will be observed.[2] Uhthoff and Loehr[3] and Speed and Hazleman[4] have commented that it is during the resorptive stage that patients are most likely to develop symptoms and this was attributed to the process of resorption of calcium itself. When osteolysis of the greater tuberosity is observed in calcific tendinopathy of the shoulder, it has been reported that there is an association with worse outcomes, more pain, more functional impairment, and less success with surgery.[16] In most cases, the pain and other symptoms will be self-limited and the natural history of the disease is for pain to improve over time without the need for aggressive interventions.

HISTORY AND PHYSICAL EXAMINATION

A complete history is important when evaluating a patient with shoulder pain. Questions to ask relate to pain with overhead activities, night pain, a history of trauma, or sports participation. It is also helpful to ask about numbness, tingling, burning, or weakness, because this may suggest a cervical radiculopathy or brachial plexopathy. A medical history significant for diabetes or thyroid disease may increase suspicion for calcific tendinopathy.

A thorough physical examination is also important when evaluating a patient with shoulder pain. The examination should begin with inspection and palpation of the painful shoulder. Active and passive range of motion of the shoulder should also be assessed. Manual muscle testing should be done to assess for weakness that may be related to pain inhibition, a rotator cuff tear, or neurologic injury. Sensation and reflexes should also be assessed if nerve damage is suspected. Finally, provocative tests should be done.

Tests classically used to assess shoulder pain related to subacromial impingement include the Hawkin impingement test, Neer sign test, and Yocum test. These maneuvers have in common the idea that when performed correctly, the subacromial space is compressed. For all of the above impingement tests, reproducible pain with the maneuver is considered a positive sign. In the Hawkin test, the shoulder is passively flexed to 90° and internally rotated by the examiner. In the Yocum test, the patient places their hand on the contralateral shoulder and elevates their elbow without elevating the shoulder in the process. The Neer sign test is performed by passively forward flexing an internally rotated shoulder.[17]

Occasionally, a patient will have constitutional symptoms of fever and malaise.[4] In these patients, elevated inflammatory markers may be found on blood work such as C-reactive protein, erythrocyte sedimentation rate, and serum white blood count.[4] In these patients, it is important to consider septic arthritis, gout, and pseudogout. Ultimately, to make the diagnosis of calcific tendinopathy of the rotator cuff, imaging studies will be needed.

IMAGING STUDIES

Plain films are often adequate to diagnose calcific tendinopathy of the rotator cuff. Anteroposterior, outlet view, internal rotation, and external rotation views are routinely ordered (**Fig. 1**). MRI can be a useful adjunct study to see if there is an associated rotator cuff tear and to evaluate for suspected osteolysis of the greater tuberosity. In addition, MRI has a distinct advantage for evaluation of the glenoid labrum, subcortical bone, and deep soft tissues when compared with other imaging modalities.

Ultrasound has become another useful tool for evaluating sources of shoulder pain, with comparable sensitivities to MRI when performed by a skilled ultrasonographer.[18,19] In addition, ultrasound allows the ultrasonographer to perform a dynamic evaluation to assess for subacromial

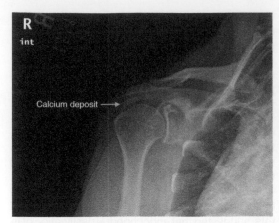

Fig. 1. Right shoulder radiograph showing large calcific deposit in the subacromial space.

impingement. Another advantage of ultrasound is that the resolution from the transducer is better than that from MRI, on the order of 200 μm with current technology.[19]

More specifically, ultrasound has been shown to be an effective tool to diagnose calcific tendinopathy and has been shown to have the ability to identify even small calcific lesions.[20] In addition, 2 separate studies showed that a positive Doppler signal within calcific deposits correlated with a patient having pain.[21,22] Clinically, this could help determine if the calcification is the cause of a patient's pain or just an incidental finding.

On ultrasound, the calcium deposits will usually have a hyperechoic appearance often with acoustic shadowing noticeable on examination (**Fig. 2**).[23] The calcification may also appear isoechoic, and an amorphous calcification will replace the normal fibrillar appearance of a tendon.[23,24] Typically, the calcifications will be found on ultrasound examination along the fibrillar-appearing tendon fibers. Frequently, they appear linearly along the tendon fiber, but may at times appear globular or amorphous if the calcification is not

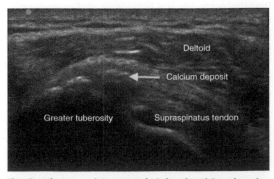

Fig. 2. Ultrasound image of right shoulder showing calcific deposit in the supraspinatus tendon.

well-formed yet.[23,24] Ultrasound may also pick up cortical bony erosions, which may help with prognosis.

TREATMENT OPTIONS
Medications

NSAIDs are a common treatment for many painful conditions. This class of medications inhibits cyclooxygenase-1 and cyclooxygenase-2 enzymes, which are important in the inflammatory cascade that produces prostaglandins and thromboxanes. They are frequently used to help treat pain associated with subacromial bursitis, rotator cuff tendonitis, and other causes of shoulder pain, including calcific tendinopathy. Although no studies have focused on what medication regimen is optimal, it is reasonable to treat patients symptomatically with NSAIDs.

Caution should always be used when prescribing NSAIDs to patients with a history of gastrointestinal or cardiac disease. Upper gastrointestinal complications, including bleeding, have been found to be increased using NSAIDs versus placebo.[25] NSAIDs, as a class, have been associated with increased risk of vascular events as well, including myocardial infarction and stroke.[25–27]

Yokoyama and colleagues[28] looked at using histamine blockade to reduce the symptoms associated with calcific tendinopathy. The rationale for using this class of medication was the decrease in serum calcium seen in patients with hyperparathyroidism treated with a histamine blocker. Sixteen patients who failed conservative treatment were treated with cimetidine for 3 months. Results showed reduced visual analog scale (VAS) scores, decreased impairment of shoulder movement, and radiologic evidence of decreased calcium deposit size compared with pretreatment. Although the mechanism is unclear, in this small sample size, cimetidine seems to have benefited these patients.

Other medications to consider include various narcotic and nonnarcotic painkillers. These medications may be considered in patients who are having difficulty sleeping secondary to moderate to severe pain.

Modalities

Multiple modalities have been used in the treatment of RCCT, including iontophoresis, therapeutic ultrasound, and extracorporal shock wave therapy (ESWT).

Acetic acid iontophoresis

Acetic acid iontophoresis (AAI) was first described in the treatment of calcific tendinosis in 1955.[29]

More recently, multiple randomized controlled trials have been performed to analyze the effectiveness of this modality. The theory is that using acetic acid will acidify the environment around the calcium depositions. Because most calcium crystals are made of hydroxyapatite crystals, the depositions should, in theory, dissolve in this environment. Iontophoresis is used to help direct the medication to deeper tissues. Two recent studies failed to show improvement with AAI in the treatment of RCCT. One study compared AAI with no treatment and found improvement in the area and density of the calcium deposits of both groups at the end of the study compared with pretreatment, but no difference between groups.[30] Similarly, Leduc and colleagues[31] found improvements in pain, range of motion, and number of calcium deposits from the beginning of the study to after the treatment period, both in those receiving AAI and in those receiving sham treatment. Time, with or without physiotherapy, seemed to improve patients' symptoms in these studies. Larger studies may be needed to show benefit, but at this time, it is difficult to recommend the use of AAI in the treatment of RCCT.

Therapeutic ultrasound

Therapeutic ultrasound may be used for painful musculoskeletal disorders and was looked at specifically in treating RCCT in one study in the *New England Journal of Medicine* in 1999. Investigators treated patients with pulsed therapeutic ultrasound for 24 sessions over a period of 6 weeks and found both decreased pain and improved quality of life when compared with sham ultrasound.[32] These results were significant at the end of the study, but the effects were no longer statistically significant at the 9-month follow-up.

Extracorporal shock wave therapy

ESWT is a modality that is often used to break up urologic calcium stones and has recently been investigated in RCCT. One group in Italy found a decrease in pain, increase in function, and associated decrease in calcium deposit size after 4 treatments with ESWT compared with sham therapy.[33] These findings were significant immediately after treatment and at 1 and 6 months after treatment.

Another study looked at long-term results for patients who received ESWT for RCCT. In this study group, most of the patients received a single treatment (n = 27), whereas others received 2 (n = 9) or 3 (n = 3) treatment sessions. At 6-month follow-up, the treatment group had decreased pain, increased power, motion, and activity when compared with the control group.[34] Calcium deposit size was also noted to be decreased in the study group, with no difference in the control group. When following these patients 2 years after treatment, 90.9% of patients had significant, if not complete, improvement in shoulder symptoms. This study, however, had a very small control group and patients were not blinded to treatment group.

Rebuzzi and colleagues[35] compared ESWT to arthroscopic surgery and found no difference between groups in functional improvement or pain reduction. No other studies that the authors are aware of directly compare nonoperative treatments to each other or to surgery.

ESWT is often not covered by insurance companies and the cost to the patient can range from $100 to $1000 per treatment session. It is often noted to be a painful procedure for patients.

Physical Therapy

The conservative management of shoulder pain related to RCCT usually involves a formal physical therapy program. Range-of-motion exercises and improving scapular mechanics can benefit patients with calcific tendinopathy. There are no available studies that outline a specific therapy protocol for patients with RCCT. However, there are many studies that look at subacromial impingement, a common sequelae of RCCT.

Scapular dyskinesis, abnormal position and movement of the scapula, can contribute to shoulder pain because of subacromial impingement.[36] Patients may feel their shoulder "catch" during abduction or flexion of the glenohumeral joint. This dynamic impingement can arise from anatomic (coracohumeral ligament thickening, calcium deposition, acromial spurring) or functional (abnormal muscle firing pattern, weak scapular stabilizers) reasons. Injury to or abnormal function of the rotator cuff muscles, which are dynamic stabilizers of the glenohumeral joint, will alter the positioning of the humeral head relative to the glenoid. Most commonly, the humerus will be more cephalad, which will decrease the subacromial space as the humerus flexes or abducts. The larger and more powerful scapular rotators, including the trapezius, rhomboids, levator scapula, latissimus dorsi, and serratus anterior, are active to varying amounts throughout scapulothoracic and glenohumeral overhead motion.[37] If these muscles are not coordinated properly in their muscle firing pattern, acromial elevation will not be adequate as the humerus rotates, which may also lead to impingement symptoms. If combining functional decreased subacromial space with a calcific deposit in the rotator cuff, the space that tendons can move under the acromion without

restriction is further reduced. Therefore, therapy should be directed at regaining optimal scapular mechanics, which will allow for better clearance of the supraspinatus tendon and subacromial bursa between the humeral head and anterior portion of the acromion.

Beneficial exercises have been identified that preferentially activate the middle trapezius, lower trapezius, and serratus anterior, with less activation of the upper trapezius.[38] These exercises can help restore proper balance of the scapular rotators. A well-organized therapy program, starting from range-of-motion and flexibility exercises, progressing to closed-chain, then open-chain, and finally sports-specific exercises, has been shown to lead to improved scapular mechanics and related shoulder pain.[39]

Injections

Various injections with differing techniques have been used in the management of RCCT. An intrabursal injection of corticosteroid may be used if the patient has symptoms of subacromial impingement and bursitis.[3] Other injection techniques attempt to address the calcium deposit more directly by breaking up and aspirating its contents.

One study used fluoroscopy to help needle guidance during aspiration and lavage of calcium deposits. They were able to aspirate calcium in 76% of the patients, and although calcium deposits were decreased in the area at 2-month follow-up, no difference was seen between patients with positive or negative aspiration of calcium.[40] Pain and range of motion were improved, although the authors questioned the clinical significance of the amount of range of motion gained.

Multiple groups have investigated lavage techniques under real-time ultrasound guidance to aspirate portions of the calcium deposits. These techniques may use 2 needles[24,41,42] or 1 needle.[43–48] The technique is often performed as follows (Figs. 3 and 4): Under ultrasound guidance, the needle is introduced in-plane with the ultrasound beam, allowing visualization of the needle throughout its path to the calcium deposit. Most investigators stress puncturing the deposit once (or twice if using the 2-needle technique) to maintain the integrity of the calcium deposit capsule and reduce calcium leakage. In the single-needle technique, once inside the calcium deposit, a small amount of fluid is injected and then pressure on the plunger is released to allow flow of calcium deposit back into the syringe. In the 2-needle technique, the second needle aspirates the introduced fluid. Often, a cloudy fluid containing calcium will

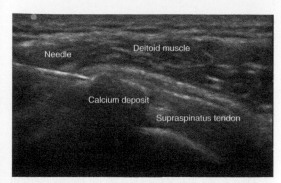

Fig. 3. Ultrasound image of right shoulder showing needle tip entering the supraspinatus calcific deposit.

be removed. This process is repeated until the aspirated fluid is clear and the calcium deposit appears smaller on ultrasound images. Once aspirated fluid is clear, or if no cloudy fluid could be removed, the deposit is needled repeatedly in an attempt to break up the remaining calcium deposit. At that point, the needle is either drawn back into the subacromial bursa or is completely withdrawn and a new needle is inserted into the subacromial bursa. A corticosteroid injection, with local anesthetic, is then administered to prevent subsequent bursitis.

Farin and colleagues[49] were the first to describe outcomes when using ultrasound guidance to perform aspiration and lavage of calcium deposits.

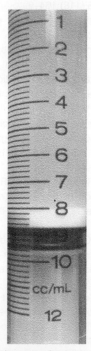

Fig. 4. Syringe with 1 mL of calcium deposit aspirated from the supraspinatus tendon.

In their 2-needle technique, they punctured the deposit 10 to 15 times before injecting saline solution, followed by aspiration of the injected fluid with a second needle until no more calcium could be removed. Results were excellent in 73% of patients and often correlated with decreased size of the deposit.

Another 2-needle technique did not include the calcium puncture before the lavage portion of the procedure. This step was omitted to maintain the cavity as intact as possible, which was assumed to facilitate more effective calcium removal. They found improved pain using both the Constant and VAS scales in the treated compared with the nontreated group at 1, 3, and 12 months after the procedure, an effect that disappeared at 5-year and 10-year follow-up.[41]

In an attempt to achieve better calcium salt dissolution, Sconfienza and colleagues[42] recently investigated the variable of saline temperature. They found shorter procedure time and easier dissolution of calcium deposits. VAS was not different between saline temperature groups, but bursitis incidence was less in warm saline-treated patients.

Other investigators use only a single needle, which further reduces the number of times the calcium cavity is violated. Bradley and colleagues[43] presented a case report of 11 patients with RCCT treated with this technique. By 2 weeks after the procedure, 10 of the patients had complete resolution of symptoms. The one patient with pain remaining had a concurrent supraspinatus tendon tear.

Yoo and colleagues[47] presented data from 35 shoulders that were treated with needle decompression via a similar technique described above. Twenty-five shoulders were almost pain free by 6 months after the procedure, and 22 experienced relief by 3 months. Six of the patients needed to undergo arthroscopic removal due because of persistent pain and were found to have rotator cuff defects at the time of surgery.

Ciampi[48] treated 50 patients with calcium deposit puncture before lavage and aspiration. At 3-month follow-up, pain was significantly improved when using the SPADI (Shoulder Pain and Disability Index) score, UCLA (University of California, Los Angeles) score, and VAS scale.[48]

At the Hospital for Special Surgery in New York, investigators retrospectively looked at 36 patients who had undergone either single-needle or double-needle aspiration followed by lavage for calcific tendinopathy. Both the numeric rating scale (NRS) score and the L'Insalata score improved after the procedure, and 77.8% of the patients rated their level of satisfaction as "good," "very good," or "excellent."[50] Four patients ended up receiving surgical treatment after the procedure.

One study investigated the difference between ESWT alone and with the addition of needling. Although both groups had improvement in Constant shoulder scores, the group who received ESWT and needling had better clinical improvement, radiologic disappearance of deposits, and less need for arthroscopic surgery.[51]

One of the limitations of many of these studies is the lack of a control group. As is well documented, calcific tendinopathy is a dynamic process that is often self-limiting, and spontaneous resorption of the deposits may occur. Comparing patients pre-procedure and after the procedure is good to track, but without a control group, it is impossible to say how much of the benefit is due to the treatment chosen or to spontaneous improvement that would have occurred without any intervention.

The specific technique used in these studies varied. A few important aspects were consistent between all of the studies:

- Calcium deposit fragmentation
- Lavage of calcium deposit with saline ± lidocaine
- Attempted aspiration of calcium.
- Subacromial bursa injection to reduce the risk of after-procedure bursitis

Although calcium removal is the goal of these procedures, it cannot always be accomplished. Ultrasound and computed tomographic images can help predict if calcific deposits will be hard and unable to aspirate or soft and able to remove calcium during needle treatment.[24] The ability to aspirate calcium may depend on the phase of the calcification,[24,43,44] and deposit type might play a role in successful treatment.[47] The ability to remove more calcium during the procedure does not result in better pain relief[42] and a decrease in calcium deposit size is seen regardless of initial ability to remove all calcium from the deposit.[43,45] Removal of calcium may not even be necessary to provide pain relief.[52]

SUMMARY

RCCT is a common finding in rotator cuff disease that can cause significant shoulder pain and disability. It usually presents as an acute tendonitis with subacromial impingement and bursitis. It can be seen easily with imaging studies such as radiography, MRI, or ultrasound. Most patients respond favorably to conservative measures. NSAIDs, modalities, and subacromial bursa steroid injections can help manage pain. Physical therapy can help improve scapular mechanics

and decrease subacromial impingement. Therapeutic ultrasound, ESWT, and ultrasound-guided needle aspiration and lavage can reduce the size of the calcium deposit and lead to substantial long-term improvement in pain and function.

REFERENCES

1. Bosworth BM. Calcium deposits in the shoulder and subacromial bursitis. J Am Med Assoc 1941; 116(22):2477–88.
2. Oliva F, Via AG, Maffulli N. Calcific tendinopathy of the rotator cuff tendons. Sports Med Arthrosc 2011;19(3):237–43.
3. Uhthoff HK, Loehr JW. Calcific tendinopathy of the rotator cuff: pathogenesis, diagnosis, and management. J Am Acad Orthop Surg 1997;5(4):183–91.
4. Speed CA, Hazleman BL. Calcific tendinitis of the shoulder. N Engl J Med 1999;340(20):1582–4.
5. Faure G, Daculsi G. Calcified tendinitis: a review. Ann Rheum Dis 1983;42(Suppl 1):49–53.
6. Oliva F, Barisani D, Grasso A, et al. Gene expression analysis in calcific tendinopathy of the rotator cuff. Eur Cell Mater 2011;21:548–57.
7. Harvie P, Pollard TC, Carr AJ. Calcific tendinitis: natural history and association with endocrine disorders. J Shoulder Elbow Surg 2007;16(2):169–73.
8. Oliva F, Via AG, Maffulli N. Physiopathology of intra-tendinous calcific deposition. BMC Med 2012;10:95.
9. Uhthoff HK, Sarkar K, Maynard JA. Calcifying tendinitis: a new concept of its pathogenesis. Clin Orthop Relat Res 1976;(118):164–8.
10. Brewer BJ. Aging of the rotator cuff. Am J Sports Med 1979;7(2):102–10.
11. Olsson O. Degenerative changes of the shoulder joint and their connection with shoulder pain; a morphological and clinical investigation with special attention to the cuff and biceps tendon. Acta Chir Scand Suppl 1953;181:1–130.
12. Mohr W, Bilger S. Basic morphologic structures of calcified tendopathy and their significance for pathogenesis. Z Rheumatol 1990;49(6):346–55 [in German].
13. Benjamin M, Rufai A, Ralphs JR. The mechanism of formation of bony spurs (enthesophytes) in the Achilles tendon. Arthritis Rheum 2000;43(3): 576–83.
14. Rui YF, Lui PP, Chan LS, et al. Does erroneous differentiation of tendon-derived stem cells contribute to the pathogenesis of calcifying tendinopathy? Chin Med J 2011;124(4):606–10.
15. Hashimoto Y, Yoshida G, Toyoda H, et al. Generation of tendon-to-bone interface "enthesis" with use of recombinant BMP-2 in a rabbit model. J Orthop Res 2007;25(11):1415–24.
16. Porcellini G, Paladini P, Campi F, et al. Osteolytic lesion of greater tuberosity in calcific tendinitis of

the shoulder. J Shoulder Elbow Surg 2009;18(2): 210–5.

17. Malanga GA, Nadler S. Musculoskeletal physical examination: an evidence-based approach. Philadelphia: Mosby; 2006.

18. Jacobson JA. Musculoskeletal ultrasound: focused impact on MRI. AJR Am J Roentgenol 2009;193(3): 619–27.

19. Levine BD, Motamedi K, Seeger LL. Imaging of the shoulder: a comparison of MRI and ultrasound. Curr Sports Med Rep 2012;11(5):239–43.

20. Papatheodorou A, Ellinas P, Takis F, et al. US of the shoulder: rotator cuff and non-rotator cuff disorders. Radiographics 2006;26(1):e23.

21. Chiou HJ, Chou YH, Wu JJ, et al. Evaluation of calcific tendonitis of the rotator cuff: role of color Doppler ultrasonography. J Ultrasound Med 2002; 21(3):289–95 [quiz: 296–7].

22. Le Goff B, Berthelot JM, Guillot P, et al. Assessment of calcific tendonitis of rotator cuff by ultrasonography: comparison between symptomatic and asymptomatic shoulders. Joint Bone Spine 2010;77(3): 258–63.

23. Jacobson JA. Fundamentals of musculoskeletal ultrasound. Philadelphia: Saunders/Elsevier; 2007.

24. Farin PU. Consistency of rotator-cuff calcifications. Observations on plain radiography, sonography, computed tomography, and at needle treatment. Invest Radiol 1996;31(5):300–4.

25. Coxib and traditional NSAID Trialists' (CNT) Collaboration, Bhala N, Emberson J, et al. Vascular and upper gastrointestinal effects of non-steroidal anti-inflammatory drugs: meta-analyses of individual participant data from randomised trials. Lancet 2013;382(9894):769–79.

26. Kearney PM, Baigent C, Godwin J, et al. Do selective cyclo-oxygenase-2 inhibitors and traditional non-steroidal anti-inflammatory drugs increase the risk of atherothrombosis? Meta-analysis of randomised trials. BMJ 2006;332(7553):1302–8.

27. Trelle S, Reichenbach S, Wandel S, et al. Cardiovascular safety of non-steroidal anti-inflammatory drugs: network meta-analysis. BMJ 2011;342: c7086.

28. Yokoyama M, Aono H, Takeda A, et al. Cimetidine for chronic calcifying tendinitis of the shoulder. Reg Anesth Pain Med 2003;28(3):248–52.

29. Psaki CG, Carroll J. Acetic acid ionization; a study of determine the absorptive effects upon calcified tendinitis of the shoulder. Phys Ther Rev 1955; 35(2):84–7.

30. Perron M, Malouin F. Acetic acid iontophoresis and ultrasound for the treatment of calcifying tendinitis of the shoulder: a randomized control trial. Arch Phys Med Rehabil 1997;78(4):379–84.

31. Leduc BE, Caya J, Tremblay S, et al. Treatment of calcifying tendinitis of the shoulder by acetic acid iontophoresis: a double-blind randomized controlled trial. Arch Phys Med Rehabil 2003;84(10):1523–7.

32. Ebenbichler GR, Erdogmus CB, Resch KL, et al. Ultrasound therapy for calcific tendinitis of the shoulder. N Engl J Med 1999;340(20):1533–8.

33. Cosentino R, De Stefano R, Selvi E, et al. Extracorporeal shock wave therapy for chronic calcific tendinitis of the shoulder: single blind study. Ann Rheum Dis 2003;62(3):248–50.

34. Wang CJ, Yang KD, Wang FS, et al. Shock wave therapy for calcific tendinitis of the shoulder: a prospective clinical study with two-year follow-up. Am J Sports Med 2003;31(3):425–30.

35. Rebuzzi E, Coletti N, Schiavetti S, et al. Arthroscopy surgery versus shock wave therapy for chronic calcifying tendinitis of the shoulder. J Orthop Trauma 2008;9(4):179–85.

36. Burkhart SS, Morgan CD, Kibler WB. The disabled throwing shoulder: spectrum of pathology Part III: The SICK scapula, scapular dyskinesis, the kinetic chain, and rehabilitation. Arthroscopy 2003;19(6):641–61.

37. Bagg SD, Forrest WJ. A biomechanical analysis of scapular rotation during arm abduction in the scapular plane. Am J Phys Med Rehabil 1988;67(6):238–45.

38. Cools AM, Dewitte V, Lanszweert F, et al. Rehabilitation of scapular muscle balance: which exercises to prescribe? Am J Sports Med 2007; 35(10):1744–51.

39. Kibler WB, McMullen J. Scapular dyskinesis and its relation to shoulder pain. J Am Acad Orthop Surg 2003;11(2):142–51.

40. Pfister J, Gerber H. Chronic calcifying tendinitis of the shoulder-therapy by percutaneous needle aspiration and lavage: a prospective open study of 62 shoulders. Clin Rheumatol 1997;16(3):269–74.

41. Serafini G, Sconfienza LM, Lacelli F, et al. Rotator cuff calcific tendonitis: short-term and 10-year outcomes after two-needle us-guided percutaneous treatment–nonrandomized controlled trial. Radiology 2009;252(1):157–64.

42. Sconfienza LM, Bandirali M, Serafini G, et al. Rotator cuff calcific tendinitis: does warm saline solution improve the short-term outcome of double-needle US-guided treatment? Radiology 2012;262(2):560–6.

43. Bradley M, Bhamra MS, Robson MJ. Ultrasound guided aspiration of symptomatic supraspinatus calcific deposits. Br J Radiol 1995;68(811):716–9.

44. Bureau NJ. Calcific tendinopathy of the shoulder. Semin Musculoskelet Radiol 2013;17(1):80–4.

45. del Cura JL, Torre I, Zabala R, et al. Sonographically guided percutaneous needle lavage in calcific tendinitis of the shoulder: short- and long-term results. AJR Am J Roentgenol 2007;189(3):W128–34.

46. Saboeiro GR. Sonography in the treatment of calcific tendinitis of the rotator cuff. J Ultrasound Med 2012; 31(10):1513–8.

47. Yoo JC, Koh KH, Park WH, et al. The outcome of ultrasound-guided needle decompression and steroid injection in calcific tendinitis. J Shoulder Elbow Surg 2010;19(4):596–600.

48. Ciampi P, Vitali M. Ultrasound-guided percutaneous needle aspiration of rotator cuff calcifications. Medicina e chirugia orthopedica 2011;1:67–9.

49. Farin PU, Rasanen H, Jaroma H, et al. Rotator cuff calcifications: treatment with ultrasound-guided percutaneous needle aspiration and lavage. Skeletal Radiol 1996;25(6):551–4.

50. Lin JT, Adler RS, Bracilovic A, et al. Clinical outcomes of ultrasound-guided aspiration and lavage in calcific tendinosis of the shoulder. HSS J 2007;3(1):99–105.

51. Krasny C, Enenkel M, Aigner N, et al. Ultrasound-guided needling combined with shock-wave therapy for the treatment of calcifying tendonitis of the shoulder. J Bone Joint Surg Br 2005;87(4):501–7.

52. Zhu J, Jiang Y, Hu Y, et al. Evaluating the long-term effect of ultrasound-guided needle puncture without aspiration on calcifying supraspinatus tendinitis. Adv Ther 2008;25(11):1229–34.

Oncology

Preface
Oncology

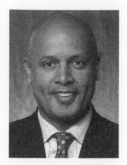

Felasfa M. Wodajo, MD
Editor

In the oncology section of this issue of *Orthopedic Clinics of North America*, we directly address the needs of nononcologic orthopedic surgeons in the evaluation of likely benign bone and soft tissue lesions.

Patients with suspected bone and soft tissue tumors can be challenging for orthopedic surgeons. While few physicians will miss the diagnosis of osteosarcoma in an adolescent with a destructive distal femur lesion, far more common is the lesion that appears benign yet still creates anxiety for the clinician and patient. However, attention to a few key imaging and clinical findings is enough to correctly diagnose five of the most common bone and soft tissue lesions.

In "Top Five Lesions That Do Not Need Referral to Orthopedic Oncology," I review the diagnostic features of lipoma, enchondroma, osteochondroma, nonossifying fibroma, and Paget disease. Accurate identification of these lesions should be within the scope of most orthopedic surgeons. As most of these patients will not need surgical treatment, referral to orthopedic oncology will not typically be required. It is hoped that this article will help guide surgeons and patients toward more expeditious resolutions for these common musculoskeletal lesions.

Felasfa M. Wodajo, MD
Musculoskeletal Tumor Surgery
Virginia Hospital Center
Orthopedic Surgery
Georgetown University Hospital
VCU School of Medicine
Inova Campus
1625 N. George Mason, Suite 464
Arlington, VA 22205-3698, USA

E-mail address:
wodajo@sarcoma.md

orthopedic.theclinics.com

Top Five Lesions That Do Not Need Referral to Orthopedic Oncology

Felasfa M. Wodajo, MD[a,b,c],*

KEYWORDS

- Lipoma • Enchondroma • Osteochondroma • Nonossifying fibroma • Paget disease • Bone biopsy
- Liposarcoma • Chondrosarcoma

KEY POINTS

- Radiography, not MRI or computed tomography, is most useful for diagnosing bone tumors.
- Most bone and soft tissue tumors have a characteristic age of presentation and radiographic appearance.
- Biopsy is not always required to diagnose many bone and soft tissue tumors.

INTRODUCTION

For many practicing orthopedic surgeons, encountering a potential bone tumor in a patient is an unwelcome challenge. Although most lesions are benign, the possibility of missing a malignancy causes understandable anxiety. Biopsy may confirm a suspected benign diagnosis but may be an unnecessary, invasive procedure in many cases, because careful analysis of clinical presentation and imaging findings will suffice for many lesions.[1] Most orthopedic surgeons are also familiar with the caveat that an inappropriately performed biopsy of a musculoskeletal malignancy may alter or harm a patient's outcome, and should be performed or guided by the treating oncologic surgeon.[2]

Many readily identifiable musculoskeletal lesions have an indolent or self-limited course and do not require treatment. Orthopedics has a built-in advantage in that x-ray, a cheap and readily available test, can often identify the underlying bone biology.[3] Some of the lesions that are identifiable on radiography include fibrous dysplasia, nonossifying fibroma, enchondroma, osteochondroma, Paget disease, and marrow infarction.[4,5]

Further, several soft tissue lesions can be reliably identified with MRI alone, including lipoma, well-differentiated liposarcoma (atypical lipoma), benign nerve sheath tumors, diffuse pigmented villonodular synovitis, fibromatosis (extra-abdominal desmoid tumor), congenital venous malformations ("intramuscular hemangioma"), and periarticular cysts (eg, Baker cysts).[6–11]

Need for Referral

Several of these lesions are indolent and sufficiently identifiable by clinical and imaging findings that routine referral to orthopedic oncology is not required.[12,13] Of course, physicians must make the appropriate decision for their patients, taking into account the clinical findings and their own training and diversity of their practice.

Five proposed lesions are as follows:

1. Lipoma
2. Enchondroma

[a] Musculoskeletal Tumor Surgery, Virginia Hospital Center, 1625 North George Mason, Suite 464, Arlington, VA 22205-3698, USA; [b] Orthopedic Surgery, Georgetown University, Washington, DC, USA; [c] Orthopedic Surgery, VCU School of Medicine, Inova Campus, VA 22205, USA
* Musculoskeletal Tumor Surgery, Virginia Hospital Center, 1625 North George Mason, Suite 464, Arlington, VA 22205-3698, USA.
E-mail address: wodajo@sarcoma.md

Orthop Clin N Am 46 (2015) 303–314
http://dx.doi.org/10.1016/j.ocl.2014.11.012

orthopedic.theclinics.com

3. Nonossifying fibroma
4. Paget disease
5. Osteochondroma

LIPOMA
Clinical Features

Lipoma is the most common neoplasm of the soft tissues.[14,15] It presents as a slowly enlarging, superficial or deep mass that has often been present for years and is most common in the proximal extremities, upper back, and abdomen. Lipomas do not diminish in size during weight loss, which sometimes leads to their discovery.

Superficial lipomas are distinctive on physical examination, presenting as soft, compressible masses with a doughy consistency. In contrast, deep lipomas may not be compressible because of the constraint of the enveloping muscle. In the absence of appropriate imaging, this may lead to unwarranted concern of a malignancy. Although superficial masses are unlikely to be painful, deep masses can be associated with activity-related symptoms.

Imaging Features

Although MRI is the gold standard for soft tissue masses, musculoskeletal ultrasound can be highly accurate in diagnosing superficial lipomas, which will appear as uniformly hypoechoic masses. When appropriately performed, ultrasound will identify the correct diagnosis for greater than 90% of superficial lipomas.[16]

On computed tomography (CT), lipomas will appear as a homogeneously low-density mass. When density is quantified on CT, lipomas will typically demonstrate negative Hounsfield units, as fat has lower density than water.[6]

Although ultrasound or CT imaging may suffice for diagnosis, MRI is always definitive. The key observation is that the appearance of the mass will be similar to that of nearby subcutaneous fat in all pulse sequences (**Fig. 1**).[6] These images should include at least a T1 and either a T2 with fat saturation or an STIR (short tau inversion recovery) sequence. Properly performed T1 images should preferably have a repetition time (TR) of less than 500 ms; values near 1000 ms are closer to proton density–weighted sequences and of less value because they also pick up water signal. Contrast administration is not required.

A special case is subcutaneous lipomas. Even grossly visible and palpable masses may not be evident on MRI, because the fat signal of the lipoma blends in with the surrounding subcutaneous fat. The combination of a visible and palpable subcutaneous mass and the absence of a mass on MRI is effectively diagnostic of a subcutaneous lipoma.

Differential Diagnosis

Although the diagnosis of lipoma, particularly with MRI, is usually straightforward, a few other lesions can have some overlapping features. Luckily, none of these poses a significant danger to the patient, and thus by extension to the diagnosing clinician.

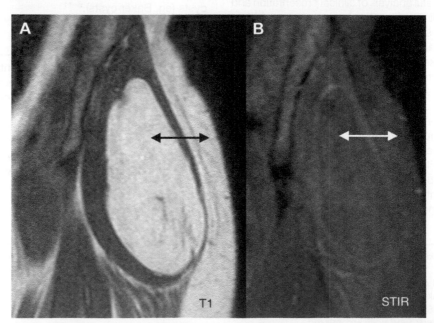

Fig. 1. Intramuscular lipoma. Thigh MRI with T1 (*A*) and fluid-sensitive short tau inversion recovery (STIR) sequences (*B*), both demonstrating identical appearance of tumor tissue to nearby subcutaneous fat (double headed arrows).

Well-differentiated liposarcoma, despite the name, has effectively no metastatic potential and low risk of recurrence with marginal excision, and is thus treated similar to lipomas. Clinically, it will typically present with more rapid growth than lipoma and is more likely to be deep-seated.[17]

The primary difference on imaging between lipoma and well-differentiated liposarcoma, also sometimes called *atypical lipoma* in the extremities, is that the latter will have more prominent septations on MRI. These appear as irregular thin lines that are low signal (dark) on T1-weighted sequences and high signal (bright) on T2-weighted sequences (**Fig. 2**). In one study,[17] experienced observers were able to correctly identify lipomas versus well-differentiated liposarcomas with 75% accuracy based on MRI alone.

Clinicians should also be aware of some common lipoma variants, including spindle-cell lipoma, which is a lipoma with a prominent fibrous component. Sometimes also called *fibrolipoma*, this is typically found as an extrafascial mass overlying the thoracic and cervical spine, mostly in men.[6] Angiolipoma is a variant often associated with pain. It is more common in the forearm and may actually represent an involuted vascular malformation.[6] In paraspinal regions, angiolipoma can be associated with radicular pain.[18] Hibernoma is a less common variant containing brown fat cells. On MRI, it contains regions with characteristic fat signal but appears more heterogeneous. It is more vascular than normal lipomas and, because it is metabolically active, will demonstrate intense uptake on positron emission tomography.[19] Lipoblastoma is a rare benign lipomatous tumor seen in children; it contains immature fat cells (lipoblasts) and is thought to later evolve into lipoma.[20]

Although not a true variant, some intramuscular lipomas will be infiltrated by traversing muscle fibers, giving a heterogeneous appearance that in some cases can be confused with well-differentiated liposarcoma.[6] However, paying attention to the correspondence between short-axis (axial) and long-axis (coronal) images should show that the heterogeneity in the fat signal is caused by traversing muscle fibers (**Fig. 3**).

Lipomatosis is a proliferative disorder of subcutaneous fat, and not a true neoplasm. The more common familial variant presents as multiple, soft, and typically painless lumps distributed throughout the trunk and proximal extremities (**Fig. 4**). It can present as early as adolescence and has an autosomal dominant transmission.[21] Multiple symmetric lipomatosis or Madelung disease is rarer, is found in the neck and face, and is associated or exacerbated by alcohol abuse.[22]

Author's Recommendation

Once lipoma is diagnosed, it is helpful to reassure the patient that lipomas do not have any malignant potential.[23] Small and asymptomatic lipomas can safely be observed. Liposuction or even steroid injections have been proposed for small superficial lipomas.[24]

Surgical treatment, if undertaken, is directed toward symptom relief and sometimes toward eliminating a large or unsightly mass. Intramuscular lipomas in particular are more likely to cause activity-related discomfort. In these cases, complete but marginal excision is adequate. Often, the lipoma will have a well-formed capsule that helps to define a clear plane between muscle and lipomatous tissue. In other instances, the lipoma will be removed in fragments. Regardless, once completely excised, lipomas rarely recur.[25]

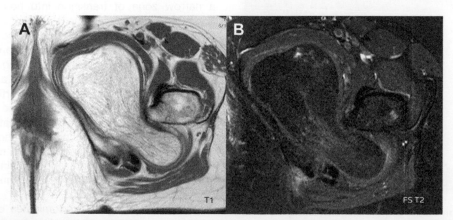

Fig. 2. Well-differentiated liposarcoma. T1 (*A*) and fat-saturated T2 MRI sequences (*B*) show a predominantly fatty mass in the deep adductor space, but with prominent septa visible on both sequences.

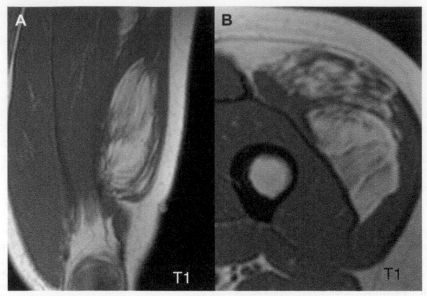

Fig. 3. Infiltrating lipoma. MRI T1 axial (*A*) and coronal (*B*) images show a fatty mass with thick traversing muscle fibers parallel to adjacent quadriceps fibers; the interspersed fibers sometimes lead to misinterpretation as liposarcoma.

ENCHONDROMA
Clinical Features

Enchondroma is the second most commonly biopsied bone tumor after osteochondroma.[5] It is the most common bone tumor in the hand, representing more than 2 of 3 lesions in one large series.[26] Enchondromas are more common in hands than feet, and very uncommon in the flat bones. Among the long tubular bones, the femur

is the most common location, followed by the humerus and tibia.[5]

The most common presentation for an enchondroma is as an incidental finding during evaluation for unrelated musculoskeletal symptoms.[27] However, in the small tubular bones of the hand and feet, enchondromas may present with pain caused by microfracture or, in up to one-third of cases, with a displaced fracture.[28]

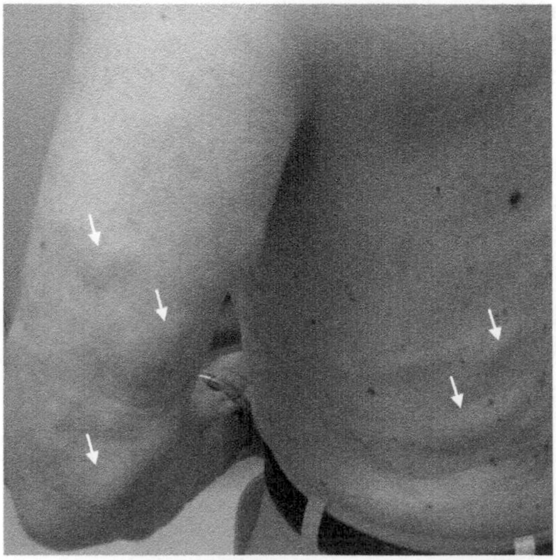

Imaging Features

Enchondromas have a characteristic appearance on radiographs, appearing as partially lytic lesions, centrally located in the metaphysis or metadiaphysis. When predominantly lytic, they demonstrate a narrow zone of transition into normal bone, consistent with their indolent nature.[5] More typically, the lesions (**Fig. 5**) will demonstrate a characteristic chondroid mineralization pattern, consisting of arcs, whorls, and stippling.[5]

In the hands, enchondromas are more commonly located in the proximal portion of the phalanges and the distal portion of the metacarpals, corresponding to the growth plates.[28] Enchondromas in the hand may not show visible mineralization on radiography, and may even show marked expansion and thinning of the cortices, in sharp contrast to the long tubular bones (**Fig. 6**).

On MRI, high signal predominates on T2 sequences, consistent with the abundant water content of cartilage. Typically, interspersed regions of

Fig. 4. Lipomatosis. Clinical image showing older patient with numerous subcutaneous nodules (*arrows*), particularly in the abdomen, flank, and upper arm.

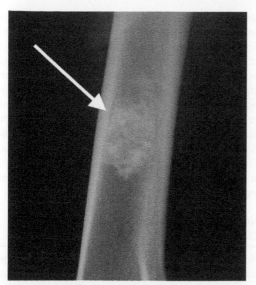

Fig. 5. Enchondroma in long bone. Typical radiographic appearance of mineralizing lesion with stippled mineralization centrally located in the metaphysis or metadiaphysis (*arrow*).

low T1 and T2 signal are present, corresponding to areas of mineralized cartilage.[28]

The extent of uptake on bone scintigraphy has been proposed to help differentiate between benign and malignant chondroid tumors, with only 21% of benign enchondromas showing more uptake than the anterior iliac spine.[29] In practice, however, scintigraphy rarely adds useful information, because most enchondromas are small, with little if any endosteal involvement, and thus easily identified as benign.

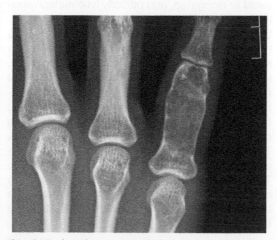

Fig. 6. Enchondroma in small bone. In the short tubular bones of the hands and feet, cortical thinning and expansion may be prominent, whereas matrix mineralization may not be visible on radiographs.

Differential Diagnosis

As the calcification that follows vascular insult to bone can demonstrate a somewhat similar stippling pattern on radiographs to that of chondroid matrix, marrow infarction can be mistaken for enchondroma. Furthermore, both conditions may be discovered in a central metaphyseal location. However, marrow infarction will often present as a longer longitudinal lesion, giving a "smoke up the chimney" appearance (**Fig. 7**).

The distinction between enchondroma and marrow infarction is more obvious if MRI is obtained, wherein the high water content of cartilage will generate a predominantly high T2 signal, which is not typically seen in marrow infarction. Enchondromas, as is typical with cartilage neoplasms, will also have a lobular growth pattern in contrast to the longitudinal, "serpiginous" pattern seen in marrow infarction. Finally, in the absence of articular surface involvement or pain, the treatment for marrow infarction is simply observation, and therefore mistaking enchondroma for marrow infarction may not be clinically significant.

However, in practice, the clinician is more often vexed in differentiating between an enchondroma and chondrosarcoma.[30] This challenge is often the result of an MRI reading suggesting that an incidentally discovered enchondroma may be a low-grade chondrosarcoma. Although some caution in the face of an unexpected finding is

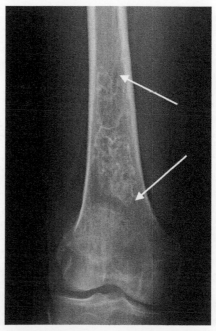

Fig. 7. Marrow infarction (*arrows*). Distal femoral lesion showing longitudinal extent and wispy, "smoke in chimney" mineralization.

prudent, this is often not a difficult distinction. Features that suggest malignancy include persistent and slowly worsening pain, large size, and deep endosteal scalloping. Overt findings of malignancy include periosteal reaction or cortical breakthrough (**Fig. 8**).[5] Chondrosarcoma is extremely uncommon in the hands and feet. Conversely, enchondroma should only be diagnosed with caution in chondroid lesions of the flat bones, like the pelvis, scapula, and ribs.

Author's Recommendation

Most incidentally discovered enchondromas can simply be observed. In clinical practice, patients typically present with regional musculoskeletal pain, which prompted the imaging studies and thus discovery of the enchondroma in the first place. In these cases, it is important to diagnose the cause of pain, at least in part to confirm that the chondroid lesion is not the source pain.[31] In some cases, intraarticular or, in the shoulder, subacromial corticosteroid injection may have a useful diagnostic role.

In most cases, the enchondroma will not fill the metaphysis, nor exhibit deep endosteal scalloping of greater than two-thirds of the cortex thickness. In the absence of these imaging findings and clinical findings that can account for the patient's symptoms, the enchondroma can simply be observed. The author's practice is to repeat the radiographs 6 and 12 months later to confirm

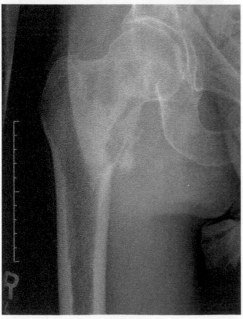

Fig. 8. Chondrosarcoma. Destructive lesion in proximal femur with stippled mineralization in the bone and adjacent soft tissue mass.

radiographic stability, during which time the patient's pain symptoms will likely have resolved. For lesions that are larger or less mineralized, noncontrast MRI may be useful to confirm the diagnosis. The author has not found technetium bone scan to be diagnostically useful, and believes it exposes patients to unnecessary radiation and anxiety. The author rarely recommends biopsy in the absence of overtly malignant features, because distinguishing between low-grade chondrosarcoma and enchondroma based on histology alone is challenging and not often helpful in decision making.

NONOSSIFYING FIBROMA
Clinical Features

Nonossifying fibroma is a very common radiologic finding, estimated to occur in up to 30% of skeletons in the first 2 decades of life.[32] In most cases, nonossifying fibroma is discovered as an incidental finding, typically in the setting of an unrelated injury leading to imaging studies. Although an uncommon cause of symptoms, large and predominantly lytic lesions in children and adolescents may be associated with activity-related pain.

Also referred to as *fibroxanthoma* or, when smaller, *cortical fibrous defects*, nonossifying fibroma is considered to be phenomenon of metaphyseal remodeling during skeletal growth rather than a true neoplastic process. The natural history is gradual reossification as the child enters the second and third decades of life.[33]

Imaging Features

Non-ossifying fibroma has a distinctive appearance on radiography, appearing as an eccentric, ovoid or elongated, and partially lytic metaphyseal lesion (**Fig. 9**). Invariably a narrow zone of transition is present between the lytic portion and the host metaphyseal bone, and sometimes a thin sclerotic interface.[34] The most common locations, in order, are distal femur, proximal tibia, proximal fibula, and distal tibia. It is uncommon in the proximal femur and proximal humerus.[32] Nonossifying fibromas are located eccentrically abutting the cortex, which may appear thinned or expanded. The exception is the fibula, where the small diameter of the bone makes the lesion appear central. The natural history of nonossifying fibromas is to reossify as the child exits the teenage years, with the portion farther away from the growth plate the first to ossify (**Fig. 10**).[12]

Differential Diagnosis

Giant cell tumors and osteosarcomas can also present as lytic metaphyseal lesions, and are

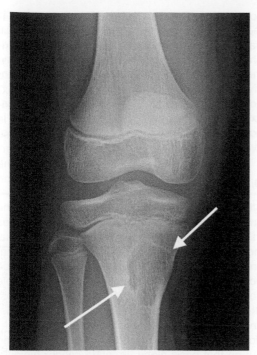

Fig. 9. Nonossifying fibroma (*arrows*). Predominantly lytic, cortically based metaphyseal lesion with thin sclerotic rim in skeletally immature patient.

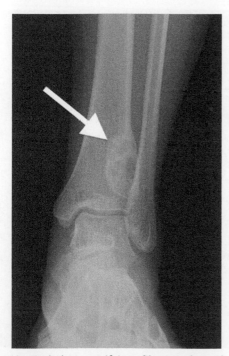

Fig. 10. Healed nonossifying fibroma (*arrow*). An eccentric metaphyseal lesion largely reossified, with the region further from growth plate more dense. Note also typical expansile cortical remodeling.

the most important conditions to exclude. Luckily, distinguishing between these and nonossifying fibromas is not often difficult based on clinical and plain radiographic findings. First, both giant cell tumors and osteosarcomas are invariably painful, whereas nonossifying fibromas most commonly present as a painless, incidental findings. Giant cell tumors are rare in the skeletally immature patient and will not demonstrate any mineralization within the lytic region. Although the involved cortex in nonossifying fibromas may be very thin, the cortical destruction of osteosarcomas will be more irregular and the medullary zone of transition will be less defined. If a partially lytic metaphyseal lesion with periosteal reaction or an adjacent mineralizing soft tissue mass is present, the diagnosis of malignancy is almost assured.

Although fibrous dysplasia and simple bone cysts may be seen in the same age group as nonossifying fibromas, their locations and appearance are different. Simple bone cysts appear as purely lytic lesions in the central metaphysis or metadiaphysis. Fibrous dysplasia is commonly found in the central diaphysis and will demonstrate a more uniform soft tissue ("ground glass") matrix.

Author's Recommendation

Most nonossifying fibromas can simply be observed. As described earlier, the radiographic findings are distinctive enough that advanced imaging is not necessary for diagnosis.[32,34] Most lesions will spontaneously heal as the child enters the third decade.[33]

The author's practice for newly discovered, asymptomatic lesions in skeletally immature patients is to repeat radiographs at 6 and 12 months, and then yearly until most of the lesion is reossified. The author has observed a few nonossifying fibromas to become more lytic and symptomatic as the child experiences a growth spurt.

For predominantly lytic lesions that occupy more than one-half the diameter of the bone and/or may be causing symptoms, referral to orthopedic oncology for possible curettage and bone grafting is appropriate.

PAGET DISEASE
Clinical Features

Paget disease is an often polyostotic disorder of bone turnover diagnosed most commonly in the pelvis. It is common in the older population, with an incidence as high as 3% to 4% in patients older than 50 years.[35] The origin is unclear, although circumstantial evidence suggests that an infectious agent may be the cause. It is most common in people of northwestern European origin and in countries largely populated by British emigrants, such as Australia and New Zealand. The prevalence of Paget disease seems to be decreasing in recent decades.[36]

Paget disease is rarely diagnosed in patients younger than 40 years. In one retrospective study, younger patients were found to be more likely to present with disease in the distal appendicular skeleton and were more likely to be African American.[37]

The most common presentation of Paget disease is of an incidental asymptomatic finding. It can also present with dull pain, not obviously related to activity. Longstanding disease may be associated in bone deformity, particularly in the tibia, or accelerated degenerative joint disease, particularly in the hip.[38] Pathologic fractures from brittle bones can occur, whereas secondary sarcoma, the most feared complication, is fortunately rare.[35]

Imaging Features

The plain radiographic findings in Paget disease are distinctive and should allow confident diagnosis in most cases. As with other metabolic and developmental conditions, the abnormalities will be longitudinally arrayed, rather than spherical or ovoid as in neoplasms. When Paget disease presents in multiple bones, the diagnosis is even clearer.

The classic findings include coarse trabeculae and thickened cortices. The affected bones may be enlarged in diameter (**Fig. 11**). The condition progresses through a predominantly lytic phase into a predominantly blastic phase, but most patients will have mixed findings.[39] In lateral radiographs of the spine, thickening of all 4 cortices gives rise to the "picture frame" appearance. The

coarsening of trabeculae in Paget disease is more pronounced than the thickened vertical trabeculae of spinal hemangiomas.[39] Delayed-phase technetium bone scan is useful in identifying the full extent of the disease and will reliably identify lesions that might be occult on radiographs.[35] Longstanding disease in the weight-bearing lower extremity bones, particularly the tibia, can result in bowing (**Fig. 12**). When severe and painful, corrective surgery for the deformity can offer relief.[38]

Differential Diagnosis

Although few skeletal conditions closely mimic the array of findings in Paget disease, some diagnoses that a clinician may consider in the differential include blastic metastatic disease, lymphoma, and fibrous dysplasia. Because Paget can be polyostotic, metastatic disease is a reasonable consideration. The primary malignancies most likely to demonstrate sclerotic changes are breast and prostate cancer, which are, of course, predominantly gender-specific and thus may be ruled out on that basis alone. Prostate cancer typically presents with numerous, discrete, small, round to ovoid blastic lesions, rather than diffuse sclerosis. Thyroid, bladder, and carcinoid cancers may also generate sclerotic skeletal metastases but are less common. Lymphoma in bone is

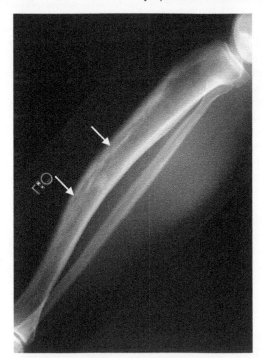

Fig. 12. Paget disease in tibia with bowing. Longstanding disease in long bone with bowing deformity, also visible is cortical thickening and "flame-shaped" intracortical lysis (*arrows*).

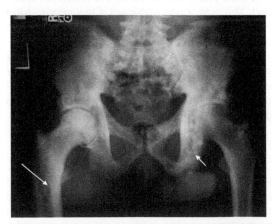

Fig. 11. Paget disease in pelvis. Diffuse involvement of pelvis and proximal femurs, demonstrating trabecular coarsening, increased diameter of ischium (short arrow), and cortical thickening (*long arrow*).

usually subtle on radiography but sometimes can also present with diffuse sclerosis. However, in none of these metastatic conditions would the dilation of bone and cortical thickening of Paget disease expect to be seen.

Similar to Paget disease, fibrous dysplasia can also be polyostotic and lead to deformity. However, the matrix is classically described as having a "ground glass," rather than sclerotic, appearance on radiographic imaging because of fibrous replacement of the marrow,[4] However, in some cases, irregular partial ossification of the fibrous tissue can produce a partially sclerotic appearance that could suggest Paget disease. The telling distinction is that, in fibrous dysplasia, broad, endosteal thinning of the cortices caused by fibrous proliferation in the marrow space is seen, in contrast to the cortical thickening of Paget disease.[4]

Author's Recommendation

The most important role of the orthopedic surgeon in Paget disease is to make the correct diagnosis, because the disease only rarely requires surgical treatment. Painful degenerative joint disease would be addressed with standard orthopedic techniques, although the increased vascularity of Pagetoid bone should be considered during total joint arthroplasty.[38] Brittle bone can lead to pathologic fracture of the subtrochanteric femur, requiring surgical treatment.[39]

Treatment of active disease is medical and based on modification of osteoclast activity, the cell primarily affected in Paget disease. Patients should be referred to endocrinology or internal medicine for bisphosphonate therapy.[40] Alkaline phosphatase and markers of bone resorption, such as urinary and serum deoxypyridinoline, N-telopeptide, and C-telopeptide, are used to identify increased bone turnover in active disease and to follow response to treatment.[38] Although calcitonin may induce remission, eventually patients develop antibodies against it.[40]

For patients with longstanding and stable Paget disease, a sudden increase in pain should alert to potential malignant transformation. In these cases, cross-sectional imaging with MRI or CT of the affected region would demonstrate a lytic destructive lesion within the Pagetoid bone. Unfortunately, the prognosis for this secondary malignancy remains dismal.[41]

OSTEOCHONDROMA
Clinical Features

Osteochondroma is often described as the most common benign bone tumor, but is really a developmental condtion rather a true neoplasm. As it constitutes 20% to 50% of all benign bone "tumors" (and 10% to 15% of all bone tumors), most orthopedic surgeons will likely encounter one or more patients with this lesion. Osteochondromas are caused by disordered bone growth at the physis, leading to bone growth perpendicular, in addition to parallel, to the longitudinal axis of the bone. Osteochondroma is the only benign bone tumor that can be caused by radiation in the growing child.[43]

Osteochondromas are not intrinsically painful. Symptoms are generally caused by irritation of the overlying tissues, typically the tendons of the adjacent joint.[44] Thus, even large sessile lesions are typically asymptomatic. Because osteochondromas are disorders of physical growth, they typically enlarge proportionally with the underlying bone until skeletal maturity. Like most bone tumors, osteochondromas are most common about the knee, with 50% occurring in the lower extremities.[42]

Hereditary multiple exostoses, as the name implies, is a heritable condition with autosomal dominant transmission that manifests with numerous osteochondromas. Like other syndromic musculoskeletal conditions, patients with multiple hereditary exostoses are diagnosed at younger ages than those with a solitary exostosis, with up to 80% discovered in the first decade of life.[45]

Imaging Features

Similar to the other lesions considered, the radiographic appearance of osteochondroma is distinctive and diagnosis can confidently be made based on plain radiography alone in most instances. Osteochondromas are exophytic lesions located juxtacortical in the metaphysis. Pedunculated lesions have a narrow base and a long stalk (**Fig. 13**). In these cases, the lesion typically points away from the nearby joint. Osteochondromas can be sessile, which appear as smooth, broad-based protuberances (**Fig. 14**).

The key in all cases is to recognize continuity of the cortex and medullary space between the host bone and the osteochondroma. This corticomedullary continuity is important in distinguishing osteochondromas from other juxtacortical lesions and tumors. In most long bone lesions, corticomedullary continuity is identifiable on radiographs, but in the flat bones such as the pelvis or scapula, cross-sectional imaging with CT or MRI may be needed to confirm the diagnosis.[42]

Differential Diagnosis

Although rare, the most concerning alternative diagnosis to osteochondroma is parosteal osteosarcoma, which is a low-grade, exophytic, surface variant of osteosarcoma. In practice, however, the

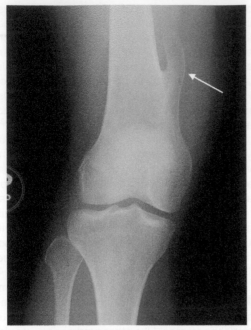

Fig. 13. Pedunculated osteochondroma (*arrow*). Typical lesion demonstrating metaphyseal location, corticomedullary continuity, and orientation away from joint.

distinction between the 2 conditions is usually straightforward. Parosteal osteosarcoma will have greater radiodensity, particularly in its more central portions, and, importantly, will not demonstrate corticomedullary continuity (**Fig. 15**). Parosteal osteosarcoma is also more commonly diagnosed later, in young adulthood. It has an excellent prognosis, with 80% to 90% survival with surgical excision alone.

Other common juxtacortical lesions are benign, and include sublingual exostosis, which is an osteochondromatous prominence of the distal

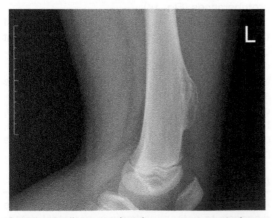

Fig. 14. Sessile osteochondroma. Juxtacortical exophytic lesion of the metaphyseal distal femur with broad base and corticomedullary continuity.

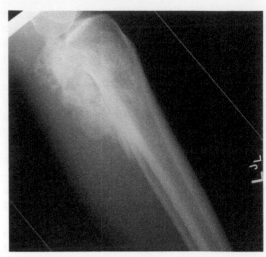

Fig. 15. Parosteal osteosarcoma. Juxtacortical exophytic metaphyseal lesion, but without corticomedullary continuity and diffuse, dense mineralization.

phalanx that causes pain and nail deformity. Nora's lesion (BPOP), or bizarre osteochondromatous proliferation, is a poorly understood, likely reactive lesion found most often in the hands and feet.[46] Periosteal chondroma is akin to an enchondroma arising from the periosteum and is more common in the proximal humerus and distal upper extremities. It presents with dull aching pain.

Author's Recommendation

Small or asymptomatic osteochondromas in skeletally mature patients can safely be ignored. In young children, the author repeats radiographs annually to observe the expected enlargement proportional with skeletal growth and monitor for musculoskeletal symptoms. In the author's experience, symptomatic lesions tend to be most common about the knee as patients enter their teens, with lesions in the lateral distal femur and the proximal medial tibia more likely to be bothersome, presumably from irritation of the distal iliotibial tract and the pes anserinus tendons, respectively.

Although transformation of solitary osteochondromas into chondrosarcoma has been reported, it is rare, with the precise rate not known but thought to be less than 1%.[42] The author's opinion is that this by itself is not indication for routine radiographic surveillance of otherwise asymptomatic osteochondromas. However, adult patients should be counseled that any change in size or symptoms around the osteochondroma should be brought to their physician's attention.

Secondary transformation is identified as a grossly thickened cartilage cap on MRI (**Fig. 16**). Most osteochondromas in adults have cartilage caps of a few millimeters. With a 2-cm cutoff,

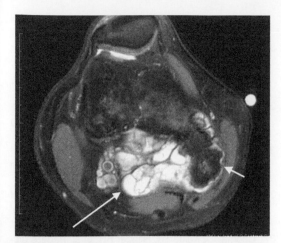

Fig. 16. Secondary chondrosarcoma. Axial, fat-saturated T2 MRI of distal femoral osteochondroma. Note appearance of normal, thin cartilage cap (*short arrow*) compared with markedly thickened, transformed cartilage (*long arrow*).

almost no secondary chondrosarcomas will be missed in adults.[47] For lesions in the distal extremities, radiographs and physical examination should be adequate to raise this suspicion. In other sites, MRI can be performed. Fortunately, the secondary chondrosarcoma in most cases is a low-grade tumor—90% in one large series—and most patients are cured with surgery alone.[48]

Children will have larger cartilage caps, typically of 1 to 3 cm. MRI does not often offer much value in pediatric patients, because transformation is rare in children.[48]

Patients with hereditary multiple exostoses would likely benefit from referral to orthopedic oncology for lifelong surveillance and management of symptoms.

SUMMARY

Although many benign skeletal neoplasms and developmental conditions can safely be observed, the conditions described herein were selected because they are both distinctive on imaging and often require no treatment. Although most orthopedic surgeons will have the experience and skills necessary to confidently diagnose these conditions, referral to orthopedic oncology colleagues remains a good option when uncertainty exists about the diagnosis or management for a particular patient. The article aims to give orthopedic surgeons the option to spare some patients anxiety-provoking and potentially unneeded referrals.

REFERENCES

1. Rougraff BT, Aboulafia A, Biermann JS, et al. Biopsy of soft tissue masses: evidence-based medicine for the Musculoskeletal Tumor Society. Clin Orthop Relat Res 2009;467(11):2783–91. http://dx.doi.org/10.1007/s11999-009-0965-9.

2. Mankin HJ, Mankin CJ, Simon MA. The hazards of the biopsy, revisited. Members of the Musculoskeletal Tumor Society. J Bone Joint Surg Am 1996;78(5):656–63.

3. Sweet D. AFIP letter Vol. 150, No. 3. archiveorg. 1992. Available at: https://archive.org/stream/AFIPLetter199206/AFIP%20Letter%201992-06_djvu.txt. Accessed July 27, 2014.

4. DiCaprio M, Enneking W. Fibrous dysplasia. Pathophysiology, evaluation, and treatment. J Bone Joint Surg Am 2005;87(8):1848–64.

5. Flemming D, Murphey M. Enchondroma and chondrosarcoma. Semin Musculoskelet Radiol 2000;4(1):59–71.

6. Murphey MD, Carroll JF, Flemming DJ, et al. From the archives of the AFIP: benign musculoskeletal lipomatous lesions. Radiographics 2004;24(5):1433–66. http://dx.doi.org/10.1148/rg.245045120.

7. McKenzie G, Raby N, Ritchie D. Non-neoplastic soft-tissue masses. Br J Radiol 2009;82(981):775–85. http://dx.doi.org/10.1259/bjr/17870414.

8. Murphey MD, Smith WS, Smith SE, et al. From the archives of the AFIP. Imaging of musculoskeletal neurogenic tumors: radiologic-pathologic correlation. Radiographics 1999;19(5):1253–80. http://dx.doi.org/10.1148/radiographics.19.5.g99se101253.

9. Murphey MD, Rhee JH, Lewis RB, et al. Pigmented villonodular synovitis: radiologic-pathologic correlation1. Radiographics 2008;28(5):1493–518. http://dx.doi.org/10.1148/rg.285085134.

10. Robbin MR, Murphey MD, Temple HT, et al. Imaging of musculoskeletal fibromatosis. Radiographics 2001;21(3):585–600.

11. Frank J, Roby C. Diagnosis, and classification of benign soft-tissue tumors. J Bone Joint Surg Am 1996;78A:126–40.

12. Wodajo FM, Gannon FH, Murphey MD. Visual guide to musculoskeletal tumors. Philadelphia: Saunders\Elsevier; 2010.

13. Ahlawat S, Blakeley J, Montgomery E, et al. Schwannoma in neurofibromatosis type 1: a pitfall for detecting malignancy by metabolic imaging. Skeletal Radiol 2013;42(9):1317–22. http://dx.doi.org/10.1007/s00256-013-1626-3.

14. Kransdorf MJ. Benign soft-tissue tumors in a large referral population: distribution of specific diagnoses by age, sex, and location. AJR Am J Roentgenol 1995;164(2):395–402. http://dx.doi.org/10.2214/ajr.164.2.7839977.

15. Myhre Jensen O. A consecutive 7-year series of 1331 benign soft tissue tumours. Clinicopathologic data. Comparison with sarcomas. Acta Orthop Scand 1981;52(3):287–93.

16. Hung EH, Griffith JF, Ng AW, et al. Ultrasound of musculoskeletal soft-tissue tumors superficial to the

investing fascia. AJR Am J Roentgenol 2014;202(6): W532–40. http://dx.doi.org/10.2214/AJR.13.11457.

17. O'Donnell PW, Griffin AM, Eward WC, et al. Can experienced observers differentiate between lipoma and well-differentiated liposarcoma using only MRI? Sarcoma 2013;2013(398):1–6. http://dx.doi.org/10.1155/2013/982784.

18. Meng J, Du Y, Yang HF, et al. Thoracic epidural angiolipoma: a case report and review of the literature. World J Radiol 2013;5(4):187–92. http://dx.doi.org/10.4329/wjr.v5.i4.187.

19. Kim JD, Lee HW. Hibernoma: intense uptake on F18-FDG PET/CT. Nucl Med Mol Imaging 2012;46(3): 218–22. http://dx.doi.org/10.1007/s13139-012-0150-z.

20. Dilley AV, Patel DL, Hicks MJ, et al. Lipoblastoma: pathophysiology and surgical management. J Pediatr Surg 2001;36(1):229–31.

21. Keskin D, Ezirmik N, Celik H. Familial multiple lipomatosis. Isr Med Assoc J 2002;4(12):1121–3.

22. Mevio E, Sbrocca M, Mullace M, et al. Multiple symmetric lipomatosis: a review of 3 cases. Case Rep Otolaryngol 2012;2012(2):1–4. http://dx.doi.org/10.1155/2012/910526.

23. Weiss SW, Goldblum JR, Folpe AL. Enzinger and Weiss's soft tissue tumors. 5th edition. Mosby (St. Louis); 2007.

24. Nanda S. Treatment of lipoma by injection lipolysis. J Cutan Aesthet Surg 2011;4(2):135–7. http://dx.doi.org/10.4103/0974-2077.85040.

25. Salam GA. Lipoma excision. Am Fam Physician 2002;65(5):901–4.

26. Simon MJ, Pogoda P, velborn FH, et al. Incidence, histopathologic analysis and distribution of tumours of the hand. BMC Musculoskelet Disord 2014;15(1): 1–8. http://dx.doi.org/10.1186/1471-2474-15-182.

27. Marco RA, Gitelis S, Brebach GT, et al. Cartilage tumors: evaluation and treatment. J Am Acad Orthop Surg 2000;8(5):292–304.

28. Larbi A, Viala P, Omoumi P, et al. Cartilaginous tumours and calcified lesions of the hand: a pictorial review. Diagn Interv Imaging 2013;94(4):395–409. http://dx.doi.org/10.1016/j.diii.2013.01.012.

29. Murphey M, Walker E, Wilson A, et al. From the archives of the AFIP: imaging of primary chondrosarcoma: radiologic-pathologic correlation. Radiographics 2003;23(5):1245–78.

30. McCarthy EF, Tyler WK. Distinguishing enchondroma from low-grade central chondrosarcoma. Pathol Case Rev 2001;6(1):8–13. http://dx.doi.org/10.1097/00132583-200101000-00003.

31. Levy J, Temple H, Mollabashy A, et al. The causes of pain in benign solitary enchondromas of the proximal humerus. Clin Orthop Relat Res 2005;431: 181–6.

32. Błaż M, Palczewski P, Swiątkowski J, et al. Cortical fibrous defects and non-ossifying fibromas in children and young adults: the analysis of radiological

features in 28 cases and a review of literature. Pol J Radiol 2011;76(4):32–9.

33. Vanel D. The incidental skeletal lesion: ignore or explore? Cancer Imaging 2009;9(Special Issue A): S38–43. http://dx.doi.org/10.1102/1470-7330.2009.9009.

34. Betsy M, Kupersmith LM, Springfield DS. Metaphyseal fibrous defects. J Am Acad Orthop Surg 2004;12(2):89–95.

35. Kaplan F, Singer F. Paget's disease of bone: pathophysiology, diagnosis, and management. J Am Acad Orthop Surg 1995;3(6):336–44.

36. Cundy T. Is the prevalence of Paget's disease of bone decreasing? J Bone Miner Res 2006;21(Suppl 2):P9–13. http://dx.doi.org/10.1359/jbmr.06s202.

37. Choma TJ, Kuklo TR, Islinger RB, et al. Paget's disease of bone in patients younger than 40 years. Clin Orthop Relat Res 2003;(418):202–4.

38. Klein GR, Parvizi J. Surgical manifestations of Paget's disease. J Am Acad Orthop Surg 2006;14(11):577–86.

39. Smith SE, Murphey MD, Motamedi K, et al. From the archives of the AFIP. Radiologic spectrum of Paget disease of bone and its complications with pathologic correlation. Radiographics 2002;22(5):1191–216.

40. Roodman GD, Windle JJ. Paget disease of bone. J Clin Invest 2005;115(2):200–8. http://dx.doi.org/10.1172/JCI24281.

41. Shaylor PJ, Peake D, Grimer RJ, et al. Paget's osteosarcoma—no cure in sight. Sarcoma 1999;3(3–4): 191–2. http://dx.doi.org/10.1080/13577149977631.

42. Murphey M, Choi J, Kransdorf M, et al. Imaging of osteochondroma: variants and complications with radiologic-pathologic correlation. Radiographics 2000;20(5):1407–34.

43. Maeda G, Yokoyama R, Ohtomo K, et al. Osteochondroma after total body irradiation in bone marrow transplant recipients: report of two cases. Jpn J Clin Oncol 1996;26(6):480–3.

44. Gitelis S, Wilkins R, Conrad EU. Benign bone tumors. Instr Course Lect 1996;45:425–46.

45. Stieber JR, Dormans JP. Manifestations of hereditary multiple exostoses. J Am Acad Orthop Surg 2005; 13(2):110–20.

46. Michelsen H, Abramovici L, Steiner G, et al. Bizarre parosteal osteochondromatous proliferation (Nora's lesion) in the hand. J Hand Surg 2004;29(3):520–5. http://dx.doi.org/10.1016/j.jhsa.2004.02.002.

47. Bernard SA, Murphey MD, Flemming DJ, et al. Improved differentiation of benign osteochondromas from secondary chondrosarcomas with standardized measurement of cartilage cap at CT and MR imaging 1. Radiology 2010;255(3):857–65. http://dx.doi.org/10.1148/radiol.10082120.

48. Ahmed AR, Tan TS, Unni KK, et al. Secondary chondrosarcoma in osteochondroma: report of 107 patients. Clin Orthop Relat Res 2003;411:193–206. http://dx.doi.org/10.1097/01.blo.0000069888.31220.2b.

Index

Note: Page numbers of article titles are in **boldface** type.

Orthop Clin N Am 46 (2015) 315–319
http://dx.doi.org/10.1016/S0030-5898(15)00025-5
0030-5898/15/$ – see front matter © 2015 Elsevier Inc. All rights reserved.

Moving?

Make sure your subscription moves with you!

To notify us of your new address, find your **Clinics Account Number** (located on your mailing label above your name), and contact customer service at:

Email: journalscustomerservice-usa@elsevier.com

800-654-2452 (subscribers in the U.S. & Canada)
314-447-8871 (subscribers outside of the U.S. & Canada)

Fax number: 314-447-8029

Elsevier Health Sciences Division
Subscription Customer Service
3251 Riverport Lane
Maryland Heights, MO 63043

Printed and bound by CPI Group (UK) Ltd, Croydon, CR0 4YY

03/10/2024

01040366-0006